Practical Approach to Diagnosis & Management of Lipid Disorders

Stephen J. Nicholls, MBBS, PhD, FRACP, FACC

Assistant Professor of Molecular Medicine
Director of Intravascular Ultrasound Core Laboratory
Clinical Director Center for Cardiovascular Diagnostics and Prevention
Cleveland Clinic
Cleveland, OH

Pia Lundman, MD, PhD, FESC

Division of Cardiovascular Medicine
Department of Clinical Sciences
Krolinska Institutet, Danderyd Hospital
Sweden

JONES AND BARTLETT PUBLISHERS

Sudbury, Massachusetts

BOSTON   TORONTO   LONDON   SINGAPORE

World Headquarters
Jones and Bartlett Publishers
40 Tall Pine Drive
Sudbury, MA 01776
978-443-5000
info@jbpub.com
www.jbpub.com

Jones and Bartlett Publishers
Canada
6339 Ormindale Way
Mississauga, Ontario L5V 1J2
Canada

Jones and Bartlett Publishers
International
Barb House, Barb Mews
London W6 7PA
United Kingdom

Jones and Bartlett's books and products are available through most bookstores and online booksellers. To contact Jones and Bartlett Publishers directly, call 800-832-0034, fax 978-443-8000, or visit our website, www.jbpub.com.

Substantial discounts on bulk quantities of Jones and Bartlett's publications are available to corporations, professional associations, and other qualified organizations. For details and specific discount information, contact the special sales department at Jones and Bartlett via the above contact information or send an email to specialsales@jbpub.com.

The authors, editor, and publisher have made every effort to provide accurate information. However, they are not responsible for errors, omissions, or for any outcomes related to the use of the contents of this book and take no responsibility for the use of the products and procedures described. Treatments and side effects described in this book may not be applicable to all people; likewise, some people may require a dose or experience a side effect that is not described herein. Drugs and medical devices are discussed that may have limited availability controlled by the Food and Drug Administration (FDA) for use only in a research study or clinical trial. Research, clinical practice, and government regulations often change the accepted standard in this field. When consideration is being given to use of any drug in the clinical setting, the healthcare provider or reader is responsible for determining FDA status of the drug, reading the package insert, and reviewing prescribing information for the most up-to-date recommendations on dose, precautions, and contraindications, and determining the appropriate usage for the product. This is especially important in the case of drugs that are new or seldom used.

Production Credits
Senior Acquisitions Editor: Alison Hankey
Senior Editorial Assistant: Jessica Acox
Production Assistant: Lisa Lamenzo
Senior Marketing Manager: Barb Bartoszek
V.P., Manufacturing and Inventory Control: Therese Connell
Composition: DiacriTech
Cover Design: Brian Moore
Cover Image: Courtesy of Dr. Cecil Fox/National Cancer Institute
Printing and Binding: Malloy, Inc.
Cover Printing: Malloy, Inc.

Library of Congress Cataloging-in-Publication Data

Nicholls, Stephen J.
    Practical approach to diagnosis & management of lipid disorders / Stephen J. Nicholls, Pia Lundman.
        p. ; cm.
    Includes bibliographical references and index.
    ISBN-13: 978-0-7637-5584-3
    ISBN-10: 0-7637-5584-2
    1. Lipids—Metabolism—Disorders. 2. Lipids—Metabolism—Disorders—Treatment. I. Lundman, Pia. II. Title. III. Title: Practical approach to diagnosis and management of lipid disorders.
    [DNLM: 1. Lipid Metabolism Disorders—diagnosis. 2. Lipid Metabolism Disorders—therapy.
WD 200.5.H8 N615p 2010]
    RC632.L5N53 2010
    616.3'997—dc22
                                                                                            2009032453

6048

Printed in the United States of America
14 13 12 11 10   10 9 8 7 6 5 4 3 2

Dedication

To Kathy, Emily, Oliver, and Angus &
Mathias, Linnéa, and Saga

Contents

Preface

For more than 100 years, it has been established that dyslipidemia plays an important role in the development of atherosclerotic cardiovascular disease. Considerable advances in risk prediction algorithms and lipid-based therapeutic strategies during the last three decades have had a profound impact on cardiovascular morbidity and mortality. At the same time, there remains a substantial residual clinical risk despite the use of conventional approaches to risk prediction and use of lipid-modifying therapies. As a result, there is considerable hope that ongoing developments and discoveries will enable more effective reduction in cardiovascular risk.

Stephen J. Nicholls
Pia Lundman

Acknowledgments

We are in debt to our mentors, colleagues, fellows, and patients who all strive to cure heart disease.

Regulation of Lipids and Their Role in Atherosclerosis

CHAPTER 1

Pathogenesis of Atherosclerosis

■ Background

- Atherosclerotic cardiovascular disease (CVD) is the leading cause of morbidity and mortality in the Western world.
- Population studies have identified a number of clinical factors that are associated with increased risk of developing atherosclerotic CVD. These include:
  - hypercholesterolemia
  - hypertension,
  - diabetes,
  - smoking,
  - low levels of HDL (high-density lipoprotein) cholesterol,
  - obesity,
  - hypertriglyceridemia, and
  - a family history of premature CVD.
- Recent reports of an association between elevated levels of inflammatory markers and prospective cardiovascular risk suggest that inflammation may also play an important role in disease promotion.
- The global spread of obesity and its associated metabolic risk factors (dyslipidemia, insulin resistance, hypertension, and inflammation) underlie projections that CVD will become the leading cause of mortality worldwide by 2020.
- The importance of an increasing prevalence of risk factors in the early stages of life is supported by findings of vascular dysfunction and evidence of macroscopic atherosclerosis in teenagers and young adults.

■ Endothelial Dysfunction

- The normal artery wall includes an endothelial layer in contact with circulating blood, underlying intima, and a medial layer. The medial layer is composed of vascular smooth muscle cells involved in the control of vascular tone and outer adventitia, which contains supporting connective tissue and the vascular and neural supply for the vessel wall itself.
- The endothelial cell layer plays an important homeostatic role regulating adhesion and migration of inflammatory cells, thrombus formation, and vascular tone. The endothelium plays a pivotal role in the synthesis and release of nitric oxide, the major mediator of its physiological functions.

- Various techniques that evaluate changes in vascular reactivity in response to factors that promote the bioavailability of nitric oxide (acetylcholine infusions, blood-pressure-cuff–induced ischemia) have been developed to assess endothelial function. These include evaluation of changes in the dimensions of conduit vessels (coronary and brachial ultrasound, flow wires) and resistance vessels (venous-strain gauge plethysmography).
- Endothelial dysfunction has been reported in association with all cardiovascular risk factors, prevalent atherosclerotic disease, and in children with a family history of premature myocardial infarction. Abnormalities of the endothelial layer are evident prior to the formation of macroscopic atherosclerotic plaque.
- Dysfunction of the endothelial layer is characterized by abnormal vascular reactivity (diminished dilatation or vasoconstriction) and expression of proinflammatory adhesion molecules (intercellular adhesion molecule-1, vascular cell adhesion molecule-1), and chemokines (monocyte chemoattractant protein-1) on the surface. Increasing expression of prothrombotic factors (von Willebrand factor) and fewer antithrombotic factors (plasminogen activator inhibitor-1, thrombomodulin) create a milieu that favors platelet adhesion and thrombus formation.

■ Formation and Propagation of Atherosclerotic Plaque

- Early histologic changes involve focal thickening of the intima with accumulation of smooth muscle cells and extracellular matrix. (See Table 1-1.) These focal changes typically occur at vascular regions associated with abnormal shear stress. Low-density lipoproteins (LDLs) diffuse into the artery wall and are trapped within the extracellular matrix by dermatan sulfate proteoglycans forming the fatty streak.
- Expression of proinflammatory adhesion molecules and chemokines on the endothelial surface promotes adhesion of circulating monocytes with subsequent migration into the intimal layer. Within the vessel wall, monocytes undergo morphologic changes to become macrophages. This is promoted by expression of the macrophage-colony-stimulating factor.
- Low-density lipoprotein undergoes chemical modification, predominantly by oxidation, within the vessel wall. Oxidized LDL is avidly taken up by macrophages via scavenger receptors. The accumulation of lipid by macrophages results in the formation of foam cells, the cellular hallmark of atherosclerotic plaque.
- The oxidation of LDL and formation of foam cells create a scenario promoting ongoing accumulation of cellular material within the artery wall. Oxidized LDL promotes further endothelial expression of proinflammatory adhesion molecules and chemokines. The foam cell also elaborates humoral factors promoting migration of lymphocytes, neutrophils, and smooth muscle cells into the artery wall.

Table 1-1:   Stages of Atherosclerosis

Endothelial dysfunction:

- Decreased nitric oxide bioavailability
- Abnormal vascular reactivity
- Expression of proinflammatory adhesion molecules and chemokines with leukocyte adhesion
- Expression of prothrombotic factors

Fatty streak formation:

- Intimal thickening
- Smooth muscle cell and extracellular matrix accumulation
- LDL trapping
- Leukocyte infiltration
- Foam cell formation

Mature plaque formation:

- Ongoing accumulation of foam cells and leukocytes
- Fibrous cap formation

Plaque rupture:

- Matrix metalloproteinase expression weakening fibrous cap
- Accumulation of necrotic core and tissue factor, which is thrombogenic
- Adventitial inflammation
- Endothelial erosion important in females and smokers

Ischemia-reperfusion injury:

- Inflammatory and oxidative mediated tissue injury with restoration of blood flow to ischemic tissue

- The accumulation of foam cells, extracellular lipid, inflammatory cells, and smooth muscle cells results in the formation of the mature atherosclerotic plaque. Collagen production by smooth muscle cells is laid down to form a fibrous cap that separates the atherosclerotic plaque from circulating blood.
- Upregulation of the expression of proteins involved in bone formation results in subsequent macroscopic calcification of atherosclerotic plaque. The development of microscopic calcific deposits, typically found within the shoulder regions, has been reported to occur in response to inflammatory stimulation.
- The artery wall has traditionally been considered a passive participant in atherosclerosis. More recent observations have demonstrated that the artery wall undergoes active changes in size and shape, termed "remodeling," in response to accumulation of atherosclerotic plaque. The typical remodeling pattern involves expansion of the outer vessel wall, with preservation of lumen dimensions. As lumen contraction occurs later in the process, substantial atherosclerosis may accumulate prior to the development of any lumen abnormalities and minor flow limitation.

■ Rupture of Atherosclerotic Plaque

■ Most atherosclerotic plaques remain clinically quiescent. The pathologic events that underlie acute ischemia involve breakdown of the integrity of the fibrous cap, bringing circulating blood into contact with plaque contents and the subsequent formation of thrombus within the arterial lumen.

■ Elaboration of metalloproteinases, which demonstrate collagenolytic and elastolytic activity, by macrophages breaks down the content and tensile strength within the fibrous cap. Histology studies reveal that rupture typically occurs in the shoulder region, associated with accumulation of macrophages and metalloproteinases.

■ A number of factors within plaque promote thrombus formation. Extracellular lipid rapidly stimulates thrombosis when exposed to blood. The thrombogenic tissue factor is produced in large quantities in plaque in response to lipid and inflammation, also rapidly promoting the coagulation cascade when plaque contents come into contact with circulating blood. The presence of necrotic material provides a further stimulus for thrombosis. The cellular contents within the plaque undergo apoptosis. Increasing intracellular contents of free cholesterol is a potent stimulator of macrophage apoptosis. As the rate of apoptosis increases to a point where it predominates over its rate of removal, the cellular debris undergoes secondary necrosis, forming a necrotic core within the plaque.

■ Initiation of thrombus formation within the arterial lumen triggers endogenous antithrombotic and fibrinolytic mechanisms to limit this process. Given the association of risk factors and atherosclerotic disease with declining levels of antithrombotic and fibrinolytic factors, the balance in favor of clot formation creates a setting where the entire lumen may become occluded, promoting acute ischemia.

■ If the balance, however, is in favor of limiting ongoing thrombus formation, then formation of another fibrous cap may seal the plaque. The potential for multiple episodes of contained plaque rupture provides an alternative mechanism for atheroma progression.

■ Ischemia-Reperfusion Injury

■ Early restoration of blood flow using fibrinolytic therapies and percutaneous intervention has been demonstrated to minimize myocardial injury and to improve the clinical outcome in patients who present with acute myocardial infarction.

■ Increasing evidence suggests that tissue reperfusion is associated with some injury. This is mediated by inflammatory and oxidative pathways. Although there has been considerable interest in the development of adjunctive therapies to minimize ischemia-reperfusion injury, none have been demonstrated to result in benefit in clinical trials.

■ Preclinical studies demonstrate that, in addition to specific anti-inflammatory and antioxidant agents, administration of HDL may limit ischemia reperfusion injury in experimental models.

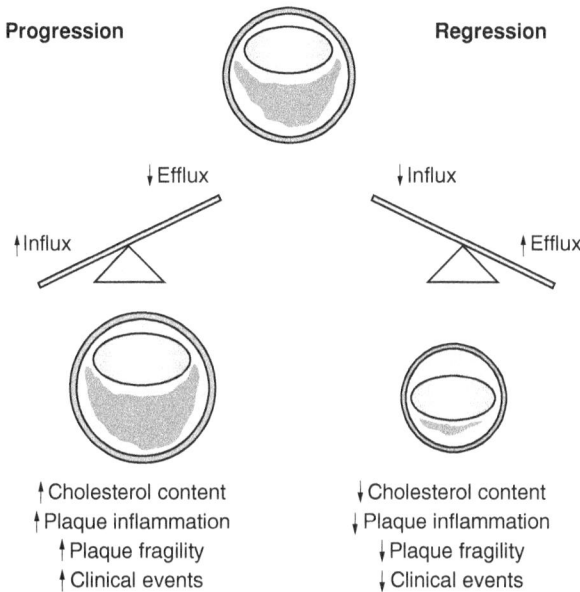

Figure 1-1: Balance between cholesterol efflux and influx and effect on pathology within the artery wall. When the scenario favors movement of cholesterol into the artery wall there is disease progression with plaque containing more lipid and inflammatory cells, generating a histologic phenotype that predisposes to plaque rupture and ischemic events. When the scenario favors movement of cholesterol out of the artery wall there is disease regression with plaque containing less lipid and inflammatory cells, generating a histologic phenotype that is less likely to undergo plaque rupture and promote acute ischemia.

■ Potential Role of Lipids in the Pathology of Atherosclerosis

■ LDL cholesterol plays a pivotal role in the formation, propagation, and rupture of atherosclerotic plaque. Although there is some evidence that small, dense LDL particles (prevalent in patients with the metabolic syndrome) may be more atherogenic, all LDL particles can have a detrimental impact on the vessel wall. (See Figure 1-1.)

■ Triglyceride-rich particles have been demonstrated to stimulate the inflammatory, oxidative, apoptotic, and thrombotic events that promote progression of atherosclerosis. This is supported by accumulating evidence from population studies that both fasting and nonfasting triglyceride levels predict prospective cardiovascular risk.

■ Lipoprotein(a) has been demonstrated to be an independent cardiovascular risk factor. The combination of an LDL particle with a discrete apolipoprotein(a) appears to be particularly atherogenic. Considerable structural homology between apolipoprotein(a) and plasminogen suggests that lipoprotein(a) may heighten the tendency to thrombus formation.

Table 1-2: Atherogenicity of Lipids

Lipid parameter	Atherogenic	Protective
Chylomicrons	+	
VLDL	+	
IDL	+	
LDL	+++	
Small, dense LDL	++++	
HDL		+++

VLDL, very low-density lipoprotein; IDL, intermediate-density lipoprotein; LDL, low-density lipoprotein; HDL, high-density lipoprotein.

- Population studies suggest that HDL cholesterol plays a protective role in atherosclerosis. Cellular and animal studies demonstrate that HDL has a beneficial effect on events participating in the formation, progression, and rupture of atherosclerotic plaque, thrombus formation, and ischemia-reperfusion injury. (See Table 1-2.)

Summary

- Accumulation of atherogenic lipids within the artery wall promote all stages of atherosclerosis from lesion formation through subsequent rupture and thrombus formation. As a result, reducing levels of atherogenic lipids is likely to have a beneficial impact on atherosclerotic cardiovascular disease.
- Increasing evidence that atherosclerosis is an inflammatory process suggests that therapeutic strategies to reduce vascular inflammation may be beneficial.
- HDLs have a number of functional properties that are likely to have a beneficial impact on the natural history of atherosclerosis.

Suggested Reading

Falk E, Shah PK, Fuster V. Coronary plaque disruption. *Circulation*. 1995;92:657–671.
Libby P. Inflammation in atherosclerosis. *Nature*. 2002;420:868–874.
Ross R. Atherosclerosis—an inflammatory disease. *N Engl J Med*. 1999;340:115–126.
Virmani R, Burke AP, Farb A, Kolodgie FD. Pathology of the unstable plaque. *Prog Cardiovasc Dis*. 2002;44:349–356.

CHAPTER 2

Metabolism of Lipids

■ Background

▣ Cholesterol and triglyceride are required by peripheral tissue for a range of homeostatic events, including the maintenance of cell membranes, synthesis of steroid hormones and bile acid, and energy utilization. Given their insolubility in plasma, these lipids are carried on a range of lipoproteins in the systemic circulation.

▣ The basic lipoprotein structure typically includes a core of esterified cholesterol and triglyceride, surrounded by a surface bilayer of phospholipid, unesterified or free cholesterol, and a range of proteins (termed "apolipoproteins").

▣ These lipoproteins differ on the basis of their size, their density, and the composition of lipid, apolipoproteins, and other factors. Not surprisingly, lipoproteins possess different functional properties in vivo. (See Table 2-1.)

▣ The major classes of lipoproteins, in order of decreasing particle size, include:
  - chylomicrons,
  - very low-density lipoprotein (VLDL),
  - intermediate-density lipoprotein (IDL),
  - low-density lipoprotein (LDL), and
  - high-density lipoprotein (HDL).

■ Metabolism of Atherogenic Lipoproteins

▣ Cholesterol enters the systemic circulation via two pathways: (1) endogenous synthesis and (2) exogenous intestinal absorption of dietary and biliary cholesterol. (See Figure 2-1.)

▣ Cholesterol, free fatty acids, and glycerol within the intestinal lumen are absorbed across the intestinal brush border into the intestinal mucosa. Within these cells, cholesterol undergoes esterification by acyl-coenzyme A:cholesterol acyltransferase (ACAT); free fatty acids and glycerol are then combined to form triglycerides. Chylomicrons are packaged within the small intestinal mucosa as particles containing predominantly triglyceride and apolipoprotein (apoB48), along with smaller amounts of apoA-I, A-II, and A-IV, and subsequently secreted into the intestinal lymphatic system.

Table 2-1: Physical Characteristics of Lipoproteins in Plasma

Lipoprotein	Lipid content	Apolipoproteins	Density (g/mL)	Diameter (A)
Chylomicron	Triglyceride	A-I, A-II, A-IV, B48, C-I, C-II, C-III, E	< 0.95	800–5000
Chylomicron remnant	Triglyceride Cholesterol ester	B48, E	< 1.006	> 500
VLDL	Triglyceride	B100, C-I, C-II, C-III, E	< 1.006	300–800
IDL	Cholesterol ester Triglyceride	B100, C-I, C-II, C-III, E	1.006–1.019	250–350
LDL	Cholesterol ester Triglyceride	B100	1.019–1.063	180–280
HDL	Cholesterol ester Triglyceride	A-I, A-II, A-IV, C-I, C-II, C-III, D	1.063–1.21	50–120

VLDL, very low-density lipoprotein; IDL, intermediate-density lipoprotein; LDL, low-density lipoprotein; HDL, high-density lipoprotein.

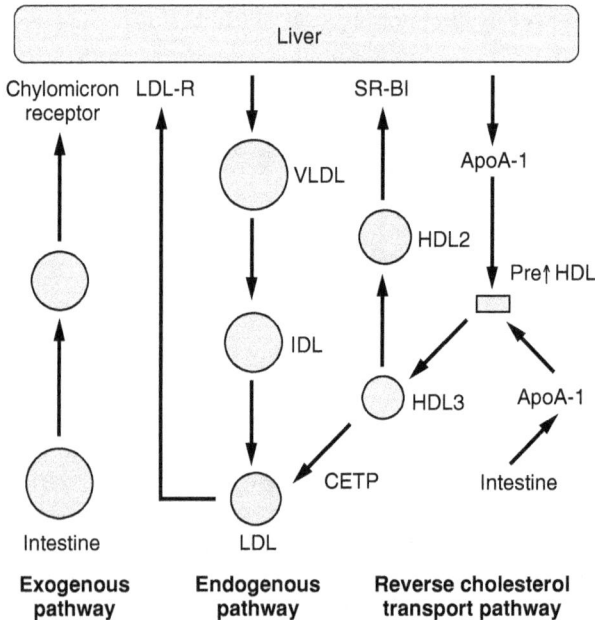

Figure 2–1: Illustrative summary of pathways involved in transportation of lipid via the exogenous, endogenous, and reverse cholesterol transport systems, which facilitates movement of cholesterol from both dietary and hepatic sources. ApoA-I, apolipoprotein A-I; CETP, cholesteryl ester transfer protein; HDL, high-density lipoprotein; IDL, intermediate-density lipoprotein; SR-BI, scavenger receptor B-I; VLDL, very low-density lipoprotein.

Interaction with HDL particles in lymph results in chylomicron enrichment with apoC-I, C-II, C-III, and E.

■ ApoC-II acts as a potent activator of lipoprotein lipase once the chylomicrons enter capillary beds, promoting hydrolysis of triglyceride to free fatty acids and generating smaller remnant particles, which contain predominantly cholesteryl ester, apoB48 and apoE. Considerable interaction takes place between chylomicrons and their remnant particles with other lipoproteins, particularly HDL, within the systemic circulation, permitting the exchange of core lipids and surface components. Remnant particles are taken up by the liver, via a receptor-mediated interaction, facilitated by apoE.

■ Endogenous lipoprotein synthesis involves production of primarily VLDL in the liver. These particles contain predominantly triglyceride and apoB100, with some esterified cholesterol and a range of additional apolipoproteins (C-II, C-III, and E). The microsomal triglyceride transfer protein factor has been identified as playing a pivotal role in providing triglyceride substrate for VLDL synthesis.

■ Upon entering the systemic circulation, VLDLs rapidly remodel by a number of processes. Activation of lipoprotein lipase by apoC-II reduces the triglyceride content and particle size, generating IDL particles. In the setting of abdominal obesity and insulin resistance, apoC-III, an inhibitor of lipoprotein lipase, tends to predominate, promoting hypertriglyceridemia. Exchange of surface components with HDL is also observed. IDLs either are taken up by the liver via a receptor-mediated process that involves apoE or are further remodeled by a lipoprotein and hepatic lipases to form LDL.

■ Further exchange of triglyceride for phospholipid and cholesteryl ester with HDL particles, promoted by phospholipid transfer protein (PLTP) and cholesteryl ester transfer protein (CETP), respectively, results in an LDL particle that contains predominantly esterified cholesterol in its core. The metabolic fate of an LDL particle involves uptake of cholesterol by cells in peripheral material or hepatic particle uptake, facilitated by the LDL receptor on the liver surface.

■ Cellular uptake of LDL particles is determined by their requirement for cholesterol. If de novo cholesterol synthesis is not adequate to meet a cell's demand, surface LDL receptor expression is increased, favoring cholesterol uptake. When a cell does not require additional cholesterol, receptor expression is reduced. Elevated systemic concentrations of LDL do have the potential to overburden a peripheral cell, whose cholesterol requirements have already been satisfied. The balance between the de novo synthetic mechanism and cell surface expression of LDL receptors has been the major target for pharmacological manipulation in order to lower levels of LDL cholesterol. Inhibiting 3-hydroxy-3-methylglutaryl coenzyme A reductase, the rate-limiting factor in cellular cholesterol synthesis, increases LDL receptor expression and therefore favors removal of LDL cholesterol from the systemic circulation.

- Lipoprotein(a) [Lp(a)] is formed extracellularly and incorporates binding of apo(a) to apoB100 on the LDL surface. A domain of apo(a) shares considerable homology with the fibrin-binding domain of the fibrinolytic factor, plasminogen. As a result, in addition to its LDL properties, Lp(a) also has the ability to inhibit thrombolysis and favor thrombus formation, further highlighting its role in the promotion of atherosclerotic cardiovascular disease.

■ Metabolism of Protective Lipoproteins

- HDLs are the smallest and most dense lipoproteins within the systemic circulation. Their basic structure similarly consists of a core of esterified cholesterol and triglycerides, surrounded by a surface bilayer of phospholipid, free cholesterol, and apolipoproteins (predominantly A-I and A-II, with small amounts of C-I, C-II, C-III, and E). The constant remodeling of HDL particles results in considerable heterogeneity in terms of their size, shape, electrophoretic mobility, and lipid composition.

- HDLs are synthesized in the liver and small intestine as lipid-free deplete particles containing phospholipid and apolipoproteins A-I, A-II, and A-IV. Interaction with other lipoprotein particles results in the rapid accumulation of other apolipoproteins: C-I, C-II, C-III, and E.

- HDL particles primarily act as acceptors of free cholesterol effluxed from cells in peripheral tissues to maintain cellular cholesterol homeostasis. It has become apparent that this transfer occurs via a number of mechanisms. Free cholesterol and phospholipid can be transferred to HDL by simple diffusion, in a concentration-gradient-guided process. Lipid-poor HDL particles are the preferential acceptors of cholesterol and phospholipid effluxed via the transmembrane protein, ATP (adenosine triphosphate) binding cassette A-1 (ABCA-1), in an energy-dependent process. The importance of ABCA-1 is highlighted by the finding that genetic deficiency of ABCA-1 underlies Tangier disease, a process characterized by excessive accumulation of intracellular cholesterol. The scavenger receptor SR-BI has been implicated in bidirectional transfer of cholesterol and phospholipid between HDL and cells. More recently, another transmembrane protein, ABCG-1, has been identified as an important pathway involved in the efflux of cholesterol from cells to mature, cholesterol-enriched HDL particles.

- Upon transfer to HDL particles, cholesterol is esterified by lecithin:cholesterol acyltransferase (LCAT), a factor activated by apoA-I. Esterified cholesterol is then stored within the particle core, maintaining a low concentration of free cholesterol on the particle surface and therefore favoring ongoing cholesterol efflux from cells. Ongoing efflux of cholesterol, initially by ABCA-1 and diffusion and then subsequently promoted by SR-BI and ABCG-1, results in the generation of large, cholesterol-rich HDL particles.

- Cholesterol within HDL particles has two metabolic fates. The traditional view holds that HDL carries its lipid contents to the liver, where it is taken up by endocytosis, facilitated by SR-BI on the liver surface. Cholesterol is removed, permitting release of the lipid-depleted HDL particle. This represents the pivotal role played by HDL in facilitation of reverse cholesterol transport, whereby excess cholesterol is removed from peripheral tissue and taken to the liver, where it is either used for synthesis of new VLDL particles or excreted in the bile.
- Alternatively, significant lipid changes within HDL particles occur in response to a range of remodeling factors in plasma. Phospholipid transfer protein (PLTP) facilitates exchange of phospholipid and triglyceride between VLDL and HDL particles. CETP facilitates exchange of triglyceride and cholesteryl ester between apoB-containing particles and HDL. Esterified cholesterol exchanged to LDL can be either taken up by the liver, providing a second pathway for reverse cholesterol transport, or delivered to cells in peripheral tissue.

■ Suggested Reading

Barter PJ. Hugh Sinclair lecture: The regulation and remodelling of HDL by plasma factors. *Atherosclerosis Suppl.* 2002;3:39–47.

Ginsberg HN. Lipoprotein physiology. *Endocrinol Metab Clin North Am.* 1998;27: 503–519.

CHAPTER 3

Genetic Lipid Abnormalities

■ Background

■ A range of familial dyslipidemic syndromes have been identified, where the primary defect is in regulation of lipoprotein synthesis or catabolism. (See Table 3-1.)

■ The familial nature of these syndromes suggests an underlying genetic etiology, which has been elucidated in some, but not all settings.

■ These syndromes are often identified by early lipid screening, with a greater prevalence in the setting of premature coronary heart disease than in the general population.

Table 3-1:   Summary of Genetic Forms of Dyslipidemia

Hypercholesterolemia:

■ Familial hypercholesterolemia
■ Familial defective apoB100
■ Polygenic hypercholesterolemia

Hypertriglyceridemia:

■ Familial hypertriglyceridemia
■ Familial hyperchylomicronemia
■ Lipoprotein lipase deficiency

HDL metabolism disorders:

■ Familial hypoalphalipoproteinemia
■ LCAT deficiency
■ Point mutations of apoA-I
■ ABCA1 deficiency

Combined hyperlipidemias:

■ Familial combined hyperlipidemia
■ Hyperapobetalipoproteinemia
■ Familial dysbetalipoproteinemia

■ Hypercholesterolemia

■ Familial hypercholesterolemia is a monogenic, autosomal dominant condition involving the defective expression and functional activity of the LDL receptor. Heterozygous deficiency is found in 1 in 500 individuals. Various phenotypes have been identified on the basis of defects in the synthesis, transportation, binding, and internalization of the receptor. This type of hypercholesterolemia is associated with severe elevation of LDL cholesterol, xanthomata, and the premature incidence of diffuse atherosclerosis. Clinical severity is greater in patients with homozygous mutations. Diagnosis is often made on the basis of severe hypercholesterolemia in the setting of normal triglyceride levels and tendon xanthomata, with a strong family history of premature coronary heart disease. Genetic and cellular studies provide confirmation of the diagnosis. Combination regimens that include high-dose statins in addition to other LDL-cholesterol-lowering agents and, on some occasions, LDL apheresis, are typically required. Accumulating evidence supports the use of intensive therapy in children and adolescents, who are deemed to be at high risk. Additional therapeutic options for resistant cases include ileal bypass or portacaval surgery, liver transplantation, and gene replacement therapy.

■ Familial defective apoB100 is an autosomal disorder involving the apoB100 ligand on the LDL receptor, resulting in similar lipid abnormalities to those observed in familial hypercholesterolemia. Clinical expression and approach to management are similar to those of heterozygous familial hypercholesterolemia.

■ Polygenic hypercholesterolemia is characterized by moderately elevated LDL cholesterol, normal triglycerides, premature atherosclerosis, and no evidence of xanthomata. Defects involving increased apoB synthesis and reduced LDL receptor expression, in addition to the presence of the apoE4 phenotype, which results in downregulation of LDL receptors, are likely to contribute to elevations in LDL cholesterol. Standard approaches to lowering LDL cholesterol are employed in these patients.

■ Hypertriglyceridemia

■ Familial hypertriglyceridemia is autosomal dominant characterized by elevated triglyceride levels, in association with insulin resistance and disordered regulation of blood pressure and uric acid levels. Underlying mutations of lipoprotein lipase promote the degree of triglyceride elevation.

■ Familial hyperchylomicronemia represents a more extensive form of lipoprotein lipase mutation, resulting in more severe hypertriglyceridemia and a milky appearance of serum.

■ Lipoprotein lipase deficiency is associated with hypertriglyceridemia, low HDL cholesterol levels, and premature atherosclerosis. In homozygous deficiency, chylomicronemia is present.

▩ In all of these settings, reduction of dietary fat consumption and initiation of triglyceride-lowering therapies are essential. Alcohol cessation, weight loss, and intensive diabetes management are required.

■ HDL Metabolism Disorders

▩ Familial hypoalphalipoproteinemia is an uncommon autosomal disorder involving mutations of the apoA-I gene and resulting in low levels of HDL cholesterol and premature atherosclerosis.

▩ Lecithin:cholesterol acyltransferase (LCAT) deficiency is characterized by defective esterification of cholesterol on the surface of HDL particles, an essential component of formation of mature HDL particles. As a result, low HDL cholesterol levels are observed, in association with corneal opacities (fish eye disease) and target cells in the presence of homozygous deficiency.

▩ Various genetic mutations of apoA-I with single amino acid substitutions have been described. The apoA-I Milano (AIM) variant has been characterized in a cohort of subjects with low HDL cholesterol levels who appear to be protected from coronary heart disease. A cysteine-for-arginine substitution in AIM permits formation of dimers and HDL particles that demonstrated efficient cholesterol efflux and anti-inflammatory activity. Infusion of reconstituted HDL particles containing AIM have a beneficial impact on lesions in animal models and promote regression of coronary atherosclerosis in humans.

▩ Tangier disease is characterized by the presence of cellular lipid accumulation with the presence of foam cells in peripheral tissues, hepatosplenomegaly, peripheral neuropathy, low levels of HDL cholesterol, and premature atherosclerosis. Mutations in ABCA1 (ATP-binding cassette A1 ABCA1) expression have been identified as the underlying defect, with impairment in cellular cholesterol efflux to lipid-deplete HDL particles, resulting in cellular cholesterol accumulation. Enhanced renal clearance of lipid-poor apoA-I promotes the reduced HDL cholesterol levels.

■ Combined Hyperlipidemias

▩ Familial combined hyperlipidemia is found in up to 2% of the population and is characterized by elevations in apoB, LDL cholesterol, and triglycerides, with differing patterns of predominance. Increased hepatic synthesis of apoB100 is the underlying defect, with relative deficiency of lipoprotein lipase activity determining the significance of hypertriglyceridemia in each individual clinical setting. Hyperapobetalipoproteinemia is a variant of familial combined hyperlipidemia in which the LDL cholesterol:apoB ratio is <1.2. Use of statins, in combination with other agents including niacin, bile acid sequestrants, ezetimibe and fibrates, depending on triglyceride levels, are typically employed.

- Familial dysbetalipoproteinemia is autosomal recessive and characterized by the presence of two apoE2 alleles, severe hypertriglyceridemia, elevated LDL cholesterol, xanthomata, and premature vascular disease. Defective clearance of VLDL and chylomicron remnants in the setting of apoE2 results in generation of dense VLDL (beta-VLDL) particles. Lipoprotein electropheresis demonstrating an elevated ratio of VLDL:triglyceride and apoE genotyping are employed for diagnosis. Given risks of vascular disease and acute pancreatitis, aggressive triglyceride lowering is required.

■ Summary

- Familial disorders of lipoprotein homeostasis result in varying degrees of hypercholesterolemia, hypertriglyceridemia, and low HDL cholesterol.
- In the majority of these syndromes, an increased risk of premature vascular disease is observed.
- Screening with a lipid profile in early adulthood is appropriate for early detection and initiation of therapy. Screening in childhood is recommended in first- and second-degree relatives.
- In many settings, refractory dyslipidemia will require use of complex regimens involving combination therapy.

■ Suggested Reading

Hachem SB, Mooradian AD. Familial dyslipidaemias: An overview of genetics, pathophysiology and management. *Drugs.* 2006;66:1949–1969.

Hovingh GK, de Groot E, van der Steeg W, et al. Inherited disorders of HDL metabolism and atherosclerosis. *Curr Opin Lipidol.* 2005;16:139–145.

Miller M, Zhan M. Genetic determinants of low high-density lipoprotein cholesterol. *Curr Opin Cardiol.* 2004;19:380–384.

Zambon A, Brown BG, Deeb SS, Brunzell JD. Genetics of apolipoprotein B and apolipoprotein AI and premature coronary artery disease. *J Intern Med.* 2006;259:473–480.

Clinical Approach to Evaluation of Patients with Lipid Disorders

CHAPTER 4

Use of Lipids in Risk Assessment

■ Background

- Population studies have established a number of major clinical factors associated with an elevated prospective risk of developing coronary heart disease. These include:
  - elevated LDL cholesterol,
  - hypertension,
  - diabetes,
  - low HDL cholesterol,
  - smoking, and
  - a family history of premature coronary heart disease.

  Increased cardiovascular risk has also been associated with the presence of obesity, hypertriglyceridemia, chronic kidney disease, and elevated levels of Lp(a).
- Accordingly, measurement of a standard lipid profile, including total cholesterol, LDL cholesterol, HDL cholesterol, and triglycerides, is recommended to form an integral component of approaches to cardiovascular risk prediction.

■ Assessment of Global Cardiovascular Risk

- Numerous risk scores have been developed to predict cardiovascular risk. These scores are based on observations of the relative degree of importance of individual major risk factors.
- The Framingham risk score (See Table 4-1.) is commonly used to predict cardiovascular risk over the next 10 years in the primary prevention setting. This score incorporates age, total cholesterol, HDL cholesterol, smoking status, systolic blood pressure, and gender. Patients can then be classified as low (<10%), intermediate (10–20%), and high (>20%) risk.
- Patients with established atherosclerotic disease are already considered to be high risk and should undergo intensive risk factor modification.
- Patients with a 10-year risk >20% (See Table 4-2.) or with diabetes are considered to be coronary heart disease risk equivalents in terms of the approach to risk factor modification.

Table 4-1: Framingham Risk Score

Parameter	Range	Points
Age (years)	20–34	–7
	35–39	–3
	40–44	0
	45–49	3
	50–54	6
	55–59	8
	60–64	10
	65–69	12
	70–74	14
	75–79	16
Total cholesterol (mg/dL)—greater weighting in younger age ranges	<160	0
	160–199	1–4
	200–239	1–8
	240–279	2–11
	>279	2–13
Smoker	Yes	1–9
HDL cholesterol (mg/dL)	>59	–1
	50–59	0
	40–49	1
	<40	2
Systolic blood pressure (mm Hg)—greater weighting if currently being treated for hypertension	<120	0
	120–129	1–3
	130–139	2–4
	140–159	3–5
	>159	4–6

Table 4-2:   Predicted 10-Year Risk According to Framingham Risk Score

10-Year risk	Points for males	Points for females
≤1	<5	<13
2–5	5–9	13–17
6–10	10–12	18–19
11–20	13–15	20–22
>20	>15	>22

■ Recommended Screening of Lipids

▦ The National Cholesterol Education Program's (NCEP) Adult Treatment Panel (ATP III) recommended that all subjects should commence screening of lipid profiles in early adulthood and that the screening should be performed every 5 years.

▦ Earlier screening in childhood and adolescence is recommended for subjects with a family history of familial dyslipidemia or premature coronary heart disease.

▦ A fasting profile that incorporates measurements of total cholesterol, LDL cholesterol, HDL cholesterol, and triglycerides is preferred to simple measurements of total cholesterol alone.

▦ There is increasing interest in the assessment of non-HDL cholesterol, total: HDL cholesterol and triglyceride:HDL cholesterol ratios, which are recommended as secondary measures for risk assessment. Determination of these parameters does not require any additional analytical measurements, and it permits a more comprehensive assessment of the total burden of atherogenic lipids and features of the atherogenic dyslipidemic state associated with obesity and the metabolic syndrome.

▦ Although accumulating evidence suggests that measurements of apolipoproteins B and A-I and lipid particle size also correlate with cardiovascular risk, it remains to be determined whether additional measurement of these factors results in incremental and cost-effective risk prediction.

▦ The relative importance of LDL cholesterol elevations in risk assessment is considered in the setting of the presence or absence of established atherosclerotic disease, coronary heart disease equivalents, and other cardiovascular risk factors.

▦ In subjects with 0–1 major cardiovascular risk factors, the LDL cholesterol goal is 160 mg/dL, with initiation of lipid-lowering therapy when the LDL cholesterol is greater than 190 mg/dL, despite lifestyle modifications. (See Table 4-3.)

- In the presence of at least two risk factors, with intermediate risk (10-year Framingham risk 10–20%), the LDL cholesterol goal is 130 mg/dL, with initiation of lipid-lowering therapy when the LDL cholesterol is greater than 160 mg/dL, despite lifestyle modifications.
- In the presence of established atherosclerotic disease or coronary heart disease equivalents (10-year Framingham risk >20%), the LDL cholesterol goal is 100 mg/dL, with initiation of lipid-lowering therapy when the LDL cholesterol is greater than 130 mg/dL, despite lifestyle modifications.
- More recently, the guidelines were amended to include an additional category with a treatment goal of 70 mg/dL for patients with established atherosclerotic disease, considered to be at very high risk. This includes patients who present with acute ischemic syndromes.
- Non-HDL cholesterol goals, corresponding to 30 mg/dL higher than LDL cholesterol goals, have also been recommended as secondary targets for risk reduction to account for the entire complement of atherogenic lipids.

Table 4-3:   Recommended Lipid Goals

Risk category	LDL cholesterol goal (mg/dL)	LDL cholesterol for lifestyle changes (mg/dL)	LDL cholesterol for drug therapy (mg/dL)	Non-HDL cholesterol goal (mg/dL)	ApoB goal (mg/dL)
Coronary heart disease at very high risk	<70	>70	>100	<100	<80
Coronary heart disease or risk equivalent (10-year >20%)	<100	>100	>130	<130	<90
2 or more risk factors					
10-year risk 10–20%	<130	>130	>130	<160	<100
10-year risk <10%	<130	>130	>160	<160	<100
0–1 risk factors	<160	>160	>190	<190	<110

■ Suggested Reading

Cooper JA, Miller GJ, Humphries SE. A comparison of the PROCAM and Framingham point-scoring systems for estimation of individual risk of coronary heart disease in the Second Northwick Park Heart Study. *Atherosclerosis*. 2005;181:93–100.

Grundy SM, Cleeman JI, Merz CN, et al. Implications of recent clinical trials for the National Cholesterol Education Program Adult Treatment Panel III guidelines. *Circulation*. 2004;110:227–239.

Grundy SM, D'Agostino RB, Mosca LJ, et al. Cardiovascular risk assessment based on US cohort studies. Findings from a National Heart, Lung, and Blood Institute workshop. *Circulation*. 2001;104:491–496.

CHAPTER 5

Evaluation of Secondary Causes of Dyslipidemia

■ Background

- A small percentage of cases with abnormal levels of LDL cholesterol, triglycerides, and HDL cholesterol are driven by concomitant medical problems and medications.
- Although relatively uncommon in lipid clinics, treatment of underlying causes typically results in reversal of lipid abnormalities.
- Accordingly, screening for secondary causes should be considered in patients assessed for dyslipidemia. (See Table 5-1.)

■ Diabetes

- Commonly associated with hypertriglyceridemia, low HDL cholesterol, and small, dense LDL particles.
- Insulin resistance, associated adiposity, increased availability of glucose and free fatty acids, and reduced activity of lipoprotein lipase are thought to drive these lipid abnormalities.
- Intensive glycemic control and reduction in abdominal adiposity can have a beneficial effect on lipid levels, particularly in the setting of hypertriglyceridemia.

■ Biliary Obstruction

- Chronic cholelithiasis and primary biliary cirrhosis are associated with hypercholesterolemia due to elevations in systemic levels of the rare lipoprotein X, with xanthomata and hyperviscosity. Relief of biliary obstruction can reverse lipid abnormalities. Although standard lipid-lowering therapies can be effectively used, statins are relatively contraindicated in patients with chronic liver disease or cholestasis. Plasmapheresis has also been employed for treatment of symptomatic xanthomata and hyperviscosity.

Table 5-1:   Secondary Causes of Hypercholesterolemia

- Hypothyroidism
- Obstructive liver disease
- Nephrotic syndrome
- Increasing consumption of saturated fat

■ Renal Disease

- Hypertriglyceridemia is commonly found in patients with chronic renal failure. This is largely due to decreased activity of lipoprotein and hepatic lipase and selective enrichment with apoC-III, each contributing to reduced hydrolysis of triglyceride-containing particles. Triglyceride abnormalities are more commonly encountered in patients treated with peritoneal dialysis, which may reflect the presence of glucose in dialysate. It has been suggested that decreased clearance of potential lipase inhibitors plays a pivotal role. Elevated levels of Lp(a) and low HDL cholesterol are also encountered and contribute to the accelerated rate of cardiovascular disease. Patients with impaired renal function are typically excluded from large clinical trials of lipid-lowering therapy, although it is currently considered that standard approaches to therapy should be adopted, even in the setting of chronic renal failure. This is particularly important given the elevated cardiovascular risk observed in patients with chronic renal failure. Careful monitoring for adverse events should be performed. (See Table 5-2.)
- Clinical trials have attempted to define the impact of lipid-lowering therapy in patients with end-stage renal failure. The Deutsche Diabetes Dialysis Study (4D) compared atorvastatin and placebo in diabetic patients with end-stage renal failure. Use of atorvastatin did not reduce the composite end point of cardiovascular mortality, nonfatal myocardial infarction, and stroke. Recently, it was reported that rosuvastatin did not reduce the incidence of cardiovascular events in patients on regular hemodialysis [an Assessment of Survival and Cardiovascular Events (AURORA)]. However, it was also noted that rosuvastatin administration was safe in these patients. The potential efficacy of lipid lowering is undergoing further investigation in the Study of Heart and Renal Protection (SHARP).
- Nephrotic syndrome is classically associated with elevated levels of LDL cholesterol, triglycerides, and Lp(a), as a result of increased hepatic apoB synthesis, due to reduced oncotic pressure and reduced catabolism of LDL and lipoprotein lipase activity. Treatment of the underlying cause of nephrotic syndrome is accompanied by improvement of lipid levels. Use of standard lipid-lowering therapies can be effective, although patients must be carefully monitored for adverse effects.

Table 5-2: Secondary Causes of Hypertriglyceridemia

- Diabetes mellitus
- Chronic renal failure
- Obesity
- Nephrotic syndrome
- Cushing syndrome
- Lipodystrophy
- HIV
- Cigarette smoking
- Excess alcohol consumption
- High-carbohydrate diets

■ Thyroid Disease

- Hypothyroidism is associated with elevated levels of LDL cholesterol and triglyceride, either in isolation or combination, with the degree of abnormality related to the extent of thyroid deficiency. Reductions in LDL receptor expression and activity, biliary cholesterol excretion, and lipoprotein lipase activity underlie the lipid abnormalities.
- Hyperthyroidism is associated with excessive activity of each of these factors and is therefore typically associated with low levels of LDL cholesterol and triglycerides.
- Given that abnormalities can be reversed with administration of thyroid replacement therapy, measurement of thyroid-stimulating hormone is recommended in the initial assessment of patients with dyslipidemia.

■ Obesity

- Abdominal obesity is associated with elevated levels of VLDL and of triglycerides and low levels HDL cholesterol.
- Weight loss, with dietary modification and diet, is associated with beneficial effects on triglyceride and HDL cholesterol levels.
- Use of endocannabinoid receptor antagonists results in reductions in weight and in waist circumference, in association with lowering triglycerides and raising HDL cholesterol.

■ Drugs

- Many concomitant medications are associated with development of dyslipidemia. As a result, initial assessment of patients with lipid abnormalities should include a comprehensive review of all pharmacologic and over-the-counter medications. (See Table 5-3.)

- Antihypertensive agents (thiazide diuretics, beta-blockers) are associated with elevated LDL cholesterol, hypertriglyceridemia, and low levels of HDL cholesterol.
- Exogenous estrogen and progestin as components of hormone replacement therapy and oral contraceptives are associated with hypertriglyceridemia and low levels of HDL cholesterol.
- Antiretroviral agents for HIV-infected patients, in particular nucleoside protease inhibitors, are associated with hypertriglyceridemia, elevated LDL cholesterol, insulin resistance, and lipodystrophy.
- Anabolic steroids, corticosteroids, cyclosporine, tamoxifen, and retinoid use are also associated with lipid abnormalities.

Table 5-3:   Drugs that Influence Lipid Levels

Drug	Elevated LDL cholesterol	Elevated triglyceride	Decreased HDL cholesterol
Thiazide diuretics	+		
Cyclosporine	+		
Amiodarone	+		
Rosiglitazone	+		
Bile acid resins		+	
Protease inhibitors		+	
Estrogen compounds		+	
Retinoids		+	
Glucocorticoids		+	
Anabolic steroids		+	
Sirolimus		+	
Beta-blockers		+	+
Progestins			+
Androgens			+

■ Summary

- Assessment of potential secondary causes of dyslipidemia should be performed when patients are initially evaluated.
- The baseline assessment of dyslipidemia should include evaluation of thyroid function, liver enzymes, fasting blood sugar, and urinalysis, in addition to careful medication history.
- Interventions directed at the underlying cause are associated with improvements in lipid levels.

■ Suggested Reading

Gau GT, Wright RS. Pathophysiology, diagnosis, and management of dyslipidemia. *Curr Probl Cardiol.* 2006;31:445–486.

Kwiterovich PO. Primary and secondary disorders of lipid metabolism in pediatrics. *Pediatr Endocrinol Rev.* 2008;5 Suppl 2:727–738.

Stone NJ. Secondary causes of hyperlipidemia. *Med Clin North Am.* 1994;78:117–141.

CHAPTER 6

Emerging Risk Markers

■ Background

■ Conventional risk prediction algorithms are based on the presence of major cardiovascular risk factors identified by population studies including:
  ● hypercholesterolemia,
  ● hypertension,
  ● diabetes,
  ● smoking,
  ● low levels of HDL cholesterol, and
  ● family history of cardiovascular disease.
■ Patients stratified as high risk (Framingham 10-year risk score >20%) require intensive risk factor modification. Patients stratified as low risk (10-year risk <10%) do not typically require pharmacological intervention but should continue to adopt lifestyle modifications (reduction of dietary fat, smoking cessation, regular exercise).
■ Intermediate-risk patients (10-year risk 10–20%) may require further investigation to categorize their cardiovascular risk.
■ Despite the use of risk prediction scores that employ these risk factors, some patients stratified as low risk experience clinical events.
■ There is a continuing effort to develop new biomarkers for improving the diagnostic accuracy of risk prediction algorithms and thus more effectively triaging the use of preventive therapies.

■ Emerging Lipid Biomarkers

■ Chemical modification of LDL is required for it to become pathogenic in the artery wall. Given that the typical mode of modification is oxidation, measurement of antibodies against oxidized forms of LDL (oxLDL) may play a role in risk stratification. Population studies have demonstrated that increasing levels of oxLDL are associated with greater cardiovascular risk. Immunization against epitopes of oxLDL is protective in animal models. Established lipid-lowering therapies predictably reduce levels of oxLDL. It remains to be determined whether oxLDL provides an incremental or greater ability to predict risk compared with measuring LDL cholesterol.

- Although triglyceride levels are obtained in most standard lipid panels, considerable debate has focused on its role in risk prediction. Increasing evidence suggests that both fasting and nonfasting triglyceride levels predict prospective cardiovascular risk. The triglyceride:HDL cholesterol ratio has become increasingly important given the prominence of mixed dyslipidemic patterns in the setting of obesity and the metabolic syndrome. A triglyceride:HDL cholesterol ratio >3.5 appears to be associated with increased cardiovascular risk.

- LDL cholesterol does not account for the entire cohort of atherogenic lipid particles within the systemic circulation. The calculation of non-HDL cholesterol has become increasingly popular because it represents the full complement of atherogenic lipids. The ATP III guidelines have included non-HDL cholesterol as a secondary target (with levels 30 mg/dL greater than the corresponding LDL cholesterol targets) for cardiovascular prevention.

- Traditional measurement of LDL and HDL cholesterol is essentially of the cholesterol carried by these lipid particles. The tests do not accurately provide a quantification specifically of the lipid particles. Quantification of apolipoprotein B (apoB) and apolipoprotein A-I (apoA-I), in contrast, provides a direct measure of the number of atherogenic and protective particles. Accordingly, they permit the ability to evaluate the particles that directly influence the accumulation of lipid within the artery wall. Levels of apoB and apoA-I have been demonstrated to predict risk and protection, accordingly, in population studies, in parallel with the findings of LDL and HDL cholesterol. The ratio of apoB:apoA-I was demonstrated to be the strongest predictor of myocardial infarction in the INTERHEART study and the strongest predictor of the benefit of statins in slowing progression of coronary atherosclerosis. Some evidence suggests that assessment of apoB and apoA-I may provide incremental risk prediction when used in place of LDL and HDL cholesterol, respectively. The cost-effectiveness of using an apolipoprotein-based approach to risk prediction has not been evaluated.

- Lipoprotein particle size and number, as determined by nuclear magnetic resonance, have been proposed as an alternative approach to evaluation of lipids in cardiovascular risk.

  - Data from population and clinical studies reveals that in subjects who experience a clinical event, despite low levels of LDL cholesterol, the number of small LDL particles is increased. As a result, the number of small LDL particles may represent an alternative or additional target for therapeutic modification of lipids.

  - Small, dense LDL particles have received increasing attention, given their relationship with the metabolic syndrome and abdominal obesity. In a similar fashion, raising the concentration of small HDL particles appeared to predict the clinical benefit of gemfibrozil on clinical events in patients with established coronary heart disease. Increasing standardization and validation of this technique will be required before it can play a role in cardiovascular risk prediction and monitoring response to therapy.

▨ The components of HDLs that contribute to their protective role remain uncertain. Interest has focused on factors in addition to the apolipoproteins carried on these particles. In particular, the paraoxonase (PON) family of enzymes, which circulates predominantly on HDL particles, is thought to play a role in the antioxidant and anti-inflammatory activities of HDL. Recent evidence has suggested that low levels of PON activity are associated with elevated systemic levels of markers of oxidative stress and with a greater likelihood of clinical events. The role of PON risk prediction requires further investigation.

■ Emerging Inflammatory Biomarkers

▨ Considerable evidence from pathology studies implies a role for inflammation in all stages of atherosclerosis from endothelial dysfunction to plaque rupture. As a result, interest has focused on the potential role of systemic markers of inflammation in predicting cardiovascular risk and in monitoring responses to therapies.

▨ C-reactive protein (CRP) is a marker of systemic inflammation, secreted mainly by the liver in response to stimulation by IL-6. Although very high levels of CRP are routinely used to measure disease activity in patients with chronic inflammatory syndromes, elevated levels of CRP detected by a high-sensitivity assay have been reported to predict cardiovascular outcome in population studies of both primary and secondary prevention. Elevated CRP levels helped to identify patients more likely to receive clinical benefit from use of pravastatin (Pravachol) in the AFCAPS/TexCAPS study. The degree of CRP lowering corresponded with lower event rates and less coronary disease progression in response to statin therapy. High-sensitivity CRP has been increasingly employed in algorithms to predict risk in addition to conventional risk factors (low <1 mg/L, intermediate 1–3 mg/L, and high >3 mg/L). The Reynolds Risk Score integrates CRP measurements in addition to traditional Framingham risk score calculations, with reports of improved risk prediction. It remains to be determined whether CRP plays a role in atherosclerosis or is simply a marker of inflammation. The cost-effectiveness of using CRP in risk prediction remains to be clarified. The Justification for the Use of Statins in Prevention: an Intervention Trial Evaluating Rosuvastatin (JUPITER) study, in which low-risk patients with an elevated CRP >2 mg/L received benefit with rosuvastatin, provides support for the concept that CRP may identify patients likely to benefit from use of preventive therapies.

▨ Myeloperoxidase (MPO) is a leukocyte-derived pro-oxidant enzyme that is released from granules of neutrophils and some lines of monocytes. A number of lines of evidence implicate an MPO role in the genesis of atherosclerosis.

MPO and its oxidant products, nitrotyrosine and chlorotyrosine, have been identified in atherosclerotic plaque and at the site of plaque rupture. MPO promotes a number of pathological events involved in plaque formation and rupture, including uptake of oxidized lipid by macrophages, impaired nitric oxide bioavailability, endothelial dysfunction, monocyte accumulation, endothelial apoptosis, and thrombus formation. MPO levels independently predict outcomes in patients presenting with acute coronary syndromes or for evaluation of chest pain of suspected cardiac etiology. MPO levels have also been demonstrated to be elevated in subjects with endothelial dysfunction.

- Lipoprotein-associated phospholipase A2 (Lp-PLA2) circulates on LDL particles and is thought to be involved in the promotion of inflammation, as a result of the release of arachidonic acid metabolites. Elevated levels of Lp-PLA2 are associated with an increased risk of cardiovascular events in studies of patients with and without established cardiovascular disease. Lp-PLA2 levels have also been demonstrated to be reduced by statins, suggesting that they may potentially be a target for therapies in addition to being used as a marker of cardiovascular risk.

- Additional biomarker assays have been developed on the basis of inflammatory mediators of the disease process. Systemic levels of adhesion molecules (VCAM-1, ICAM-1), chemokines (MCP-1), and cytokines (IL-1, TNF-α) have been reported in some, but not all, studies to predict cardiovascular outcome. The true incremental value of these markers in the setting of conventional risk factor assessment remains to be defined.

■ Other Emerging Biomarkers

- Abdominal obesity is associated with a dramatic increase in cardiovascular risk. This is likely to result from the interaction of metabolic risk factors (hypertriglyceridemia, low HDL cholesterol, small dense LDL, insulin resistance, hypertension, and inflammation). It has also become apparent that abdominal adipose cells elaborate a range of factors, termed adipocytokines. These factors have effects on metabolic regulation and directly on the artery wall. As a result, it has been proposed that adipocytokines may predict cardiovascular risk. Elevated levels of leptin and resistin are both associated with an adverse cardiovascular outcome. In contrast, adiponectin, which appears to have a favorable influence on a number of pathological events in the artery wall, predicts relative protection from cardiovascular disease. As the prevalence of abdominal obesity increases worldwide, the potential utility of these factors is likely to be more extensively investigated.

- Each of the pathological pathways involved in the generation and subsequent rupture of atherosclerotic plaque might theoretically reveal systemic markers that may be of utility in risk prediction and in monitoring the response to therapy.

- Additional markers of oxidative stress may be of utility. The lack of use of any marker of oxidative stress complicates the assessment of the apparent lack of efficacy of reportedly antioxidant vitamins in large clinical trials. Systemic levels of the MPO products, chlorotyrosine and nitrotyrosine, predict risk and are reduced in association with statin therapy. Various metabolites of arachidonic acid can be measured in both blood and urine and have been reported as associated with cardiovascular risk. Particular care is necessary to reduce artificial oxidation at the time of specimen collection and handling.
- Breakdown of collagen integrity within the fibrous cap is a major event preceding fibrous cap rupture. Elevated levels of metalloproteinases (MMP) and reduced levels of their tissue inhibitors (TIMPs) have been reported in association with elevated cardiovascular risk in some studies. Favorable effects on these systemic factors have been reported in association with statin therapy. It remains to be determined whether MMP activity would provide effective risk stratification.
- Thrombus formation within the artery lumen is the pivotal event that promotes luminal compromise. Systemic levels of factors involved in regulation of thrombosis have been reported to predict cardiovascular risk. Elevated levels of prothrombotic factors, tissue factor, and von Willebrand factor, as well as reduced levels of protective factors, PAI-1, and thrombomodulin, have been reported in association with a greater risk of cardiovascular events in studies. Homocysteine is a factor involved in the promotion of both thrombosis and inflammation. Although lowering levels of homocysteine with folic acid has not been demonstrated to be protective in clinical trials, elevated systemic levels do correlate with cardiovascular risk, suggesting that it does play an important role in disease pathogenesis. Platelet-derived microparticles may play an important role in the regulation of thrombotic and inflammatory events. Their role in risk prediction is currently the source of investigation. Measures of platelet activity have also been reported to be of use by some groups, although standardization of these assays has been difficult to achieve.

■ Future Markers of Risk

- Noninvasive arterial wall imaging permits the discovery of subclinical atherosclerosis. These techniques have been employed to evaluate the potential efficacy of therapeutic agents. The potential utility of these modalities to predict risk and therefore subsequently to alter or monitor therapy has not been systematically investigated in large clinical trials. The potential to integrate traditional risk factors with both emerging biomarkers and atherosclerosis imaging is a field that continues to expand.
- The role of genetics in cardiovascular disease continues to become apparent. Genetic profiling of large population cohorts is currently in progress to identify new markers of risk and novel targets for therapeutic modification.

The potential of genotyping to tailor therapy in individuals remains a hypothesis in need of exploration.

■ Summary

■ A large number of novel biomarkers that reflect a broad range of pathological events involved in the progression of atherosclerosis has been reported in association with cardiovascular risk.

■ Assessment of global risk may require integration of multiple biomarkers reflecting the different pathological pathways involved in atherosclerosis.

■ The ability of these factors to provide incremental risk prediction, to tailor therapy, or to monitor the effects of therapy in a cost-effective manner remains to be determined in large clinical trials.

■ Suggested Reading

Ballantyne CM, Hoogeveen RC, Bang H, et al. Lipoprotein-associated phospholipase A2, high-sensitivity C-reactive protein, and risk for incident coronary heart disease in middle-aged men and women in the Atherosclerosis Risk in Communities (ARIC) study. *Circulation*. 2004;109:837–842.

Ballantyne CM, Nambi V. Markers of inflammation and their clinical significance. *Atheroscler Suppl*. 2005;6:21–29.

Bansal S, Buring JE, Rifai N, Mora S, Sacks FM, Ridker PM. Fasting compared with nonfasting triglycerides and risk of cardiovascular events in women. *JAMA*. 2007;298:309–316.

Bittner V, Johnson BD, Zineh I, et al. The triglyceride/high-density lipoprotein cholesterol ratio predicts all-cause mortality in women with suspected myocardial ischemia: A report from the Women's Ischemia Syndrome Evaluation (WISE). *Am Heart J*. 2009;157:548–555.

Brennan ML, Penn MS, Van Lente F, et al. Prognostic value of myeloperoxidase in patients with chest pain. *N Engl J Med*. 2003;349:1595–1604.

Lerman A, McConnell JP. Lipoprotein-associated phospholipase A2: A risk marker or a risk factor? *Am J Cardiol*. 2008;101:11F–22F.

Maki KC, Galant R, Davidson MH. Non-high-density lipoprotein cholesterol: The forgotten therapeutic target. *Am J Cardiol*. 2005;96:59K–64K; discussion 34K–35K.

Nicholls SJ, Hazen SL. Myeloperoxidase and cardiovascular disease. *Arterioscler Thromb Vasc Biol*. 2005;25:1102–1111.

Ridker PM. Clinical applications of C-reactive protein for cardiovascular disease detection and prevention. *Circulation*. 2003;107:363–369.

Ridker PM, Buring JE, Rifai N, Cook NR. Development and validation of improved algorithms for the assessment of global cardiovascular risk in women: The Reynolds Risk Score. *JAMA*. 2007;297:611–619.

Ridker PM, Buring JE, Shih J, Matias M, Hennekens CH. Prospective study of C-reactive protein and the risk of future cardiovascular events among apparently healthy women. *Circulation*. 1998;98:731–733.

Ridker PM, Cannon CP, Morrow D, et al. C-reactive protein levels and outcomes after statin therapy. *N Engl J Med*. 2005;352:20–28.

Ridker PM, Cushman M, Stampfer MJ, Tracy RP, Hennekens CH. Inflammation, aspirin, and the risk of cardiovascular disease in apparently healthy men. *N Engl J Med*. 1997;336:973–979.

Ridker PM, Rifai N, Clearfield M, et al. Measurement of C-reactive protein for the targeting of statin therapy in the primary prevention of acute coronary events. *N Engl J Med*. 2001;344:1959–1965.

Ridker PM, Rifai N, Pfeffer MA, Sacks F, Braunwald E. Long-term effects of pravastatin on plasma concentration of C-reactive protein. The Cholesterol and Recurrent Events (CARE) Investigators. *Circulation*. 1999;100:230–235.

Ridker PM, Rifai N, Pfeffer MA, et al. Inflammation, pravastatin, and the risk of coronary events after myocardial infarction in patients with average cholesterol levels. Cholesterol and Recurrent Events (CARE) Investigators. *Circulation*. 1998;98:839–844.

Tsimikas S, Brilakis ES, Miller ER, et al. Oxidized phospholipids, Lp(a) lipoprotein, and coronary artery disease. *N Engl J Med*. 2005;353:46–57.

Tsimikas S, Willerson JT, Ridker PM. C-reactive protein and other emerging blood biomarkers to optimize risk stratification of vulnerable patients. *J Am Coll Cardiol*. 2006;47:C19–C31.

Therapeutic Approach to Lipid Disorders

CHAPTER 7

Approaches to Lipid Modification

■ Background

■ As evidence has accumulated in support of the role of lipids in the pathogenesis of atherosclerotic cardiovascular disease, there has been an immense search to develop approaches to lower systemic levels of atherogenic lipids and to promote the protective properties of HDL.

■ The last 5 decades have witnessed the development of a vast range of dietary, pharmacological, and nutritional supplements that have had varying effects on lipid levels.

■ The finding that a number of these strategies have reduced the incidence of cardiovascular events in large, prospective clinical trials has led to their widespread use in therapeutic guidelines for reduction of cardiovascular risk. (See Table 7-1.)

Table 7-1: Major Classes of Lipid-Modifying Therapies

Therapeutic class	LDL cholesterol	Triglyceride	HDL cholesterol	Comments
Statins	↓ 20–55%	↓ 15–35%	↑ 3–15%	Established clinical benefit in primary and secondary prevention. Beneficial effects on atherosclerosis progression. Nonlipid lowering properties may contribute to benefit.
Fibrates	↓ 5–20%	↓ 20–50%	↑ 5–20%	Relatively weak PPAR-α (peroxisome proliferator-activated receptor) agonists increasing transcription of HDL apolipoproteins and factors promoting reverse cholesterol transport. Anti-inflammatory properties may also be important. Variable effect of individual agents in clinical trials. Concomitant administration of gemfibrozil (Lopid) associated with higher rate of myopathy with statins.

Table 7-1:   Continued

Therapeutic class	LDL cholesterol	Triglyceride	HDL cholesterol	Comments
Bile acid sequestrants	↓ 10–25%	↑ 0–10%	↑ 3–5%	Potential increase in triglyceride levels. Often limited by GI intolerance.
Niacin	↓ 15–25%	↓ 20–50%	↑15–35%	Most effective HDL-raising drug with beneficial effects on clinical events and atherosclerosis progression. Effective lowering of Lp(a). Emerging developments aim to reduce flushing and allow more patients to achieve clinically effective high doses.
Ezetimibe	↓ 15–20%	↓ 0–10%	↑0–5%	Cholesterol absorption inhibitor. Incremental lowering of CRP when administered in combination with statin therapy.
Fish oils	↑ 3–5%	↓ 30–40%	No change	Primarily used in hypertriglyceridemic patients. Lipid benefit may contribute to efficacy in clinical trials.

■ Statins

- Statins are the most commonly used agents for reduction of LDL-C and prevention of cardiovascular disease.
- They competitively inhibit 3-hydroxy-3-methylglutaryl-coenzyme A reductase (HMG CoA reductase), the rate-limiting step in endogenous cholesterol synthesis, by blocking the binding site for substrates. Consequent upregulation of the LDL receptor on the liver surface further reduces systemic LDL-C levels by up to 60%.
- Decreased hepatic synthesis of VLDL particles and increased uptake via the LDL receptor result in concomitant reductions in triglyceride levels by 15% to 35%.
- HDL-C levels increase by up to 15% as a result of a combination of an increase in hepatic synthesis of apoA-I, decreased apoA-I catabolism, and reduced CETP activity, primarily due to reduced substrate availability.

- Greater lowering of LDL-C and triglycerides are observed with later generation statins (atorvastatin, rosuvastatin). The most dramatic effect on HDL-C levels is observed with use of rosuvastatin.
- The impact of genetic factors on the disposition and effect of statins continues to be elucidated but is clearly significant. Variability in drug metabolism and expression of HMG CoA reductase may influence effects on LDL-C levels and the incidence of side effects. Genetic variability is likely to underscore the observation that Eastern Asian patients typically require very small statin doses to achieve a lipid-lowering effect.
- Increasing evidence suggests that statins also possess off-target or pleiotropic properties, beyond their effects on HMG CoA reductase, which may contribute to their cardiovascular benefit. Inhibition of protein isoprenylation by statins has been demonstrated to have favorable effects on inflammatory, oxidative, proliferative, and apoptotic pathways involved in atherosclerosis. These in vitro effects have been largely observed with high statin concentrations. These effects may be particularly important in contributing to the early benefit of statins in patients with acute coronary syndromes.
- Numerous reports from observational studies have suggested that statins may also have a beneficial impact on development of diabetes, bone density and osteoporotic bone fractures, blood pressure, and risk of dementia and cancer. However, none of these findings has been substantiated in large clinical trials or meta-analyses.
- Given the widespread administration of statins, significant attention has focused on potential adverse effects, particularly on muscle, liver, and kidneys. Of interest, adverse effects are more commonly encountered with use of lipophilic (lovastatin, fluvastatin, simvastatin, atorvastatin) than with use of hydrophilic (pravastatin, rosuvastatin) agents. (See Table 7-2.)

Table 7-2: Clinical Factors that Predispose to Muscle Adverse Side Effects with Statins

- Age (elderly patients)
- Sex (females)
- Renal impairment
- Hepatic dysfunction
- Hypothyroidism
- Corticosteroid use
- Polypharmacy
- Chronic alcohol excess
- Use of lipophilic statins
- Use of cytochrome P450 3A4 metabolizers

- The effect of statins on muscles spans a spectrum including asymptomatic creatine kinase (CK) elevations, myalgia, myositis, and rhabdomyolosis. Muscle events are more commonly observed in predisposed patients who are elderly or who are associated with chronic alcohol consumption, renal failure, cholestatic liver disease, hypothyroidism, or use of concomitant medical therapies that inhibit cytochrome P450 3A4 activity.

- CK rises and myalgia are found in up to 10% of patients. These are not typically associated with any long-term effects and are rapidly reversible upon discontinuation of drug therapy. Although CK levels are typically measured at baseline and with the development of muscular symptoms, routine monitoring during the course of therapy is not typically advocated. Alternative causes for CK elevations should be sought, particularly in the asymptomatic patient.

- Upon discontinuation of therapy, rechallenge should be considered, particularly with pravastatin and fluvastatin, which are associated with less muscle toxicity.

- The interest in myopathic complications has been reinforced by its incidence in patients treated with the combination of statins with fibric acid derivatives. Cerivastatin was removed from the market because it led to serious rhabdomyolysis, when used in combination with statin therapy. Muscular effects are more commonly observed when gemfibrozil, compared with fenofibrate, is used in combination with statin therapy.

- Depletion of ubiquinone (coenzyme Q10) has been proposed as a factor involved in the generation of myalgia and myopathy in statin-treated patients. Although coadministration of coenzyme Q10 has been proposed as a means to reduce the likelihood of muscle problems, this has not been tested in robust prospective clinical trials. (See Figure 7-1.)

- Dose-dependent elevations in liver transaminases are observed in up to 3% of patients. There is currently no convincing evidence of progression to hepatitis or hepatic injury. The use of routine monitoring of liver enzymes in statin-treated patients is controversial. Although some physicians monitor liver enzymes at baseline and within 12 weeks of initiation or dose escalation, monitoring is reserved by other physicians for use only in patients with liver disease or use of concomitant medications that increase systemic statin levels.

- Inhibition of renal tubular protein absorption results in benign proteinuria with statin therapy. Despite some episodes of renal impairment observed with rosuvastatin 80 mg, a dose that has been discontinued, there is no convincing data of significant renal failure with use of any available statin at currently available doses. This finding has been confirmed from patient registries, large clinical trials, and meta-analyses.

- Statins are contraindicated in pregnancy and in women who are trying to conceive due to reports of neurological and limb abnormalities associated with use of lipophilic agents in the first trimester.

Acetyl-CoA

↓

Acetoacetyl-CoA

↓

HMG-CoA

↓ *HMG-CoA reductase*

Mevalonate

↓

Gernayl pyrophosphate

↓

Farnesyl pyrophosphate ⟶ Polyprenyl pyrophosphate

Squalene synthase ↓

Squalene

↓

Ubiquinone (coenzyme Q10)   Cholesterol   Geranylgeranyl pyrophosphate

Protein isoprenylation

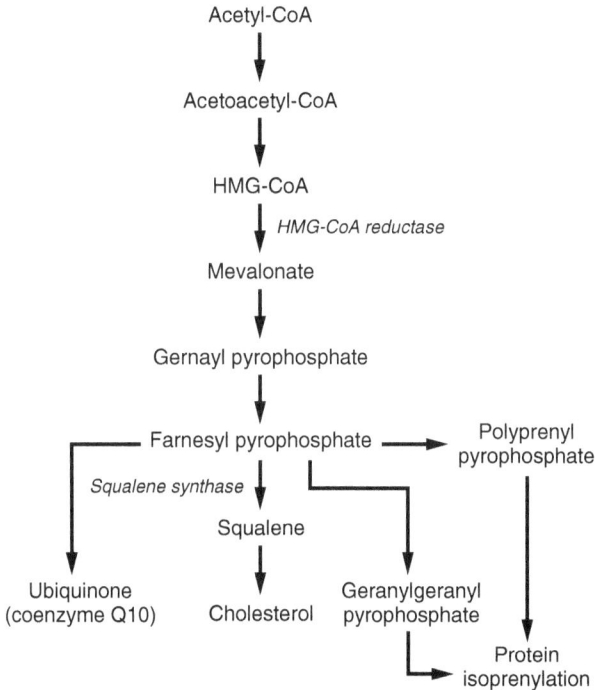

Figure 7-1: Synthetic pathway leading to the endogenous generation of cholesterol with the rate-limiting step involving the conversion of hydroxymethylglutaryl coenzymeA (HMG-CoA) to mevalonate. Steps catalyzed by HMG-CoA reductase and squalene synthase have been developed as therapeutic strategies to reduce cholesterol synthesis.

▪ Observations from small studies have also suggested that statin use may be associated with worsening of depression, increased suicide risk, hemorrhagic strokes, memory loss, cancer, peripheral neuropathy, and cataracts. Large clinical trials and meta-analyses have failed to confirm the relationship between statin use and any of these effects.

▪ Fibric Acid Derivatives (Fibrates)

▪ Fibrates act predominantly as weak pharmacologic agonists of peroxisome proliferator-activated receptor (PPAR-α), ubiquitously expressed nuclear hormone receptors.

▪ The predominant lipid effects involve reductions in triglyceride levels by 35% to 50% as a result of reduced hepatic VLDL synthesis and stimulated activity of lipoprotein lipase. HDL-C levels are increased by 5% to 20% due predominantly to enhanced hepatic expression of apoA-I and apoA-II. Several other factors involved in reverse cholesterol transport, including LCAT and SR-BI (scavenger receptor BI), are also stimulated by fibrates. Variable effects on levels of Lp(a) are also observed.

- Effects beyond lipids include reductions in fibrinogen and uric acid and elevations in homocysteine levels. Their impact on overall cardiovascular risk is unknown.
- Muscle toxicity is particularly important when fibrates are used in combination with statins. Patients taking fibrates and statins should be monitored carefully. Drug interactions should be considered particularly in patients treated with cyclosporine and warfarin.

■ Bile Acid Sequestrants

- Bile acid sequestrants are long-standing agents used to reduce levels of LDL-C either as monotherapy by up to 25% or in combination with statins or niacin.
- Inhibition of enterohepatic cycling of cholesterol by binding intestinal bile acids and subsequent upregulation of hepatic LDL receptor expression reduce LDL-C levels.
- They are poorly tolerated by many patients due to gastrointestinal symptoms, including nausea and bloating. Reversible liver transaminase elevations are observed in some patients. Careful monitoring of impaired drug absorption (warfarin, digoxin, fat-soluble vitamins) should be considered.

■ Nicotinic Acid (Niacin)

- Niacin has multiple lipid effects. It inhibits hepatic VLDL synthesis, resulting in reductions of LDL-C by up to 25%. It is the most effective, raising HDL-C by up to 35%, as a result of delayed apoA-I catabolism and inhibition of lipid exchange between VLDL and HDL particles. The effects on HDL-C levels are often observed at lower doses than those required to lower LDL-C. Lp(a) levels are also reduced by up to 35% when used at high doses.
- Many patients are unable to achieve high enough doses for effective modification of lipid levels due to flushing and pruritis. Various strategies have been employed to minimize this, including the use of a very slow dose escalation strategy, avoidance of caffeine, and pretreatment with low-dose aspirin, with variable effect. The early promise that extended-release forms would be better tolerated still has to be convincingly demonstrated. The identification of interaction between niacin and prostanoid receptors on epidermal Langerhans cells provides a mechanism underlying niacin-induced flushing. Administration of niacin preparations in combination with prostanoid receptor antagonists is currently under investigation in clinical trials.

▪ Niacin is associated with a number of additional metabolic effects, including:
  • elevation of glucose, uric acid, and homocysteine levels and lowering of blood pressure in patients treated with vasodilators.
▪ As a result, care should be taken with regard to use in patients with diabetes or gout. Liver transaminase elevations are commonly encountered, with rare episodes of hepatotoxicity reported. As a result, monitoring of liver enzymes is advised.

▪ Ezetimibe

▪ Ezetimibe impairs intestinal absorption of cholesterol at the level of the brush border, in a mechanism that is likely to involve modification of the protein Niemann-Pick C1.
▪ It lowers LDL-C by up to 20% when used as monotherapy and by 15% when used in combination with other lipid-lowering therapies. Unlike bile acid sequestrants, ezetimibe has no effect on triglyceride levels or absorption of fat-soluble vitamins.
▪ Generally well tolerated, it has been proposed as a strategy to minimize statin doses. However, this approach has not been demonstrated in clinical trials to reduce cardiovascular events.
▪ Anecdotal episodes of myalgia, rhabdomyolysis, hepatitis, pancreatitis, and thrombocytopenia have been reported.

▪ Fish Oils

▪ Fish oils are omega-3 polyunsaturated fatty acids, including eicosapentanoic acid (EPA) and docosahexaenoic acid (DHA), that are found in many food sources, particularly fleshy fish. They are thought to be one of the major factors underlying observations that populations reporting high dietary intakes of fish are associated with relative protection from cardiovascular disease.
▪ Lipid effects involve predominantly lowering of triglyceride levels as a result of reductions in hepatic synthesis of apoB and VLDL particles. In addition, reduced particle remodeling tends to result in less small, dense LDL particles. Fish oils do not typically have any effect on HDL-C levels.
▪ Fish oils have a number of additional properties that are likely to contribute to their cardiovascular benefit, including favourable effects on blood pressure, membrane stability, activation of the coagulation pathway, and endothelial function.
▪ The major intolerance involves eructation and a fishy aftertaste, both of which appear to be less problematic with more recent preparations.
▪ It is unknown whether generation of lipid peroxide species or reductions in vitamin E levels have any clinical effect.
▪ These observations underscore dietary guidelines that recommend regular consumption of fish. Extradietary supplementation is typically reserved for patients with hypertriglyceridemia.

■ Additional Strategies

■ Plant sterols/stanols competitively inhibit intestinal cholesterol absorption. Compensatory upregulation of hepatic LDL receptor expression further decreases systemic LDL-C levels. The poor water solubility of these compounds requires that they be incorporated with other compounds, such as fatty acids in margarines and salad dressings. Consumption of sterol-enriched margarine can reduce LDL-C by 15% compared with use of nonfortified margarines. Generous portions are required, and such fortified margarines are significantly more expensive than nonfortified types.

■ Various food components have been reported to have some effect on lipid levels. Isoflavones within soy products can reduce LDL-C and prevent LDL oxidation, although modest effects are observed even with use of relatively high amounts. It is likely that the reduction in saturated fat intake that parallels soy consumption is of greater importance in providing any cardiovascular benefit, compared with effects on LDL-C. Claims that garlic and plant extracts, such as guggul and policosanol, can reduce LDL-C have not been validated in large clinical trials. Interestingly, red yeast rice contains monacolins, which inhibit HMG CoA reductase and therefore lower LDL-C levels. Diets enriched with nuts and fiber are also associated with reductions in LDL-C, further supporting their inclusion in dietary guidelines for cardiovascular prevention. Furthermore, lowering LDL-C is one of the mechanisms that underlie the potential protective influence of extracts from green tea.

■ Suggested Reading

Burnett JR, Huff MW. Cholesterol absorption inhibitors as a therapeutic option for hypercholesterolaemia. *Expert Opin Investig Drugs*. 2006;15:1337–1351.

Chen ZY, Jiao R, Ma KY. Cholesterol-lowering nutraceuticals and functional foods. *J Agric Food Chem*. 2008;56:8761–8773.

Davidson MH. The use of colesevelam hydrochloride in the treatment of dyslipidemia: A review. *Expert Opin Pharmacother*. 2007;8:2569–2578.

Davidson MH, Robinson JG. Lipid-lowering effects of statins: A comparative review. *Expert Opin Pharmacother*. 2006;7:1701–1714.

Kamanna VS, Ganji SH, Kashyap ML. Niacin: An old drug rejuvenated. *Curr Atheroscler Rep*. 2009;11:45–51.

Rosenson RS. Fenofibrate: Treatment of hyperlipidemia and beyond. *Expert Rev Cardiovasc Ther*. 2008;6:1319–1330.

Skulas-Ray AC, West SG, Davidson MH, Kris-Etherton PM. Omega-3 fatty acid concentrates in the treatment of moderate hypertriglyceridemia. *Expert Opin Pharmacother*. 2008;9:1237–1248.

Staels B, Maes M, Zambon A. Fibrates and future PPARalpha agonists in the treatment of cardiovascular disease. *Nat Clin Pract Cardiovasc Med*. 2008;5:542–553.

CHAPTER 8

LDL Cholesterol

■ Background

- Low-density lipoprotein particles are found within the systemic circulation. The particles comprise of a core of esterified cholesterol, surrounded by a surface bilayer of phospholipid, apoB-100, and small amounts of free cholesterol.
- Cholesterol is derived from cellular and dietary sources. It is produced endogenously from its substrate, acetate, via a complex series of enzymatic steps. The rate-limiting step of endogenous cholesterol synthesis involves the generation of mevalonic acid, in a step catalyzed by 3-hydroxy-3-methylglutaryl coenzyme A reductase (HMGCoA reductase). Cholesterol is also absorbed via the small intestine, where it appears in the systemic circulation in apoB48-containing chylomicron particles. LDL particles are derived from the remodeling of VLDLs and IDLs in the systemic circulation. VLDLs are synthesized in the liver as particles containing triglyceride, small amounts of cholesterol, phospholipids, and apoB-100. Rapid interaction with other lipid particles and remodeling factors in the circulation results in the generation of smaller, higher-density LDL particles, containing a greater amount of esterified cholesterol in the core.
- LDL is a major transporter of cholesterol in the circulation to peripheral tissues, where the cholesterol is used for maintenance of cell membranes. LDL particles are taken up by the liver, via an interaction with the LDL receptor. Cholesterol is either reutilized for lipoprotein formation or excreted in the bile. Enterohepatic recycling of cholesterol in the terminal small intestine ensures that some biliary cholesterol is reabsorbed.
- LDL particles readily migrate into the artery wall and become trapped by proteoglycans and undergo oxidative modification. Oxidized LDL is readily taken up by arterial wall macrophages, stimulating plaque formation. Small LDL particles are considered by many to be particularly atherogenic, given their relative ease in migrating into the artery wall and susceptibility to undergoing oxidation. Accordingly, LDL cholesterol has received considerable interest in the pathogenesis of atherosclerosis and as a therapeutic target to reduce cardiovascular risk.

■ Population Studies

■ Early pathology examination of atherosclerotic plaque revealed the presence of cholesterol crystals, suggesting that dyslipidemia played a significant role in the disease process.

■ Early studies revealed lipemic blood in patients with atherosclerotic cardiovascular disease. Subsequent population studies demonstrated a curvilinear relationship between levels of both total and LDL cholesterol and prospective cardiovascular risk. The Framingham study revealed that in a population cohort of subjects without established clinical cardiovascular disease, each 1% increase in LDL cholesterol is associated with a 1% increase in cardiovascular risk.

■ Patients with hereditary disorders of cholesterol metabolism have an increased risk of cardiovascular disease. Familial hypercholesterolemia, which is associated with a defect in LDL receptor activity and as a result with very high levels of LDL cholesterol, is accompanied by a dramatic increase in premature cardiovascular disease. Angiographic studies have revealed the presence of extensive and diffuse disease in patients with familial hypercholesterolemia.

■ Subsequent studies have revealed that measurement of apoB, LDL particle size and number, and oxLDL may provide some incremental role in risk stratification.

■ Animal Studies

■ There are early findings that cholesterol feeding induced formation of atherosclerotic lesions in rabbits. These observations were subsequently supported in mouse models following genetic deletion of either apoE or the LDL receptor. More recent studies have observed that long-term cholesterol supplementation generates a histologic phenotype including lipid, inflammatory cells, and necrotic material.

■ Administration of oxidized LDL in cellular models results in foam cell formation, proinflammatory, and prothrombotic effects. Loading macrophages with free cholesterol promotes apoptosis.

■ Restoration of cholesterol-fed animals to a chow diet is accompanied by slowing of disease progression, promotion of regression, and generation of a more stable plaque phenotype, characterized by a reduction in lipid and inflammatory material and an increase in smooth muscle cells and fibrous tissue.

■ Pharmacological intervention with lipid-lowering strategies, such as statins, is associated with a beneficial impact on both the extent and composition of experimental atherosclerosis.

■ A major limitation of cholesterol-fed animal models of atherosclerosis is their lack of spontaneous plaque rupture. Rupture has traditionally been provoked by measures including catecholamine administration or balloon injury within plaque. A number of recent reports have described animal cohorts with a relatively high incidence of plaque rupture. Some groups suggest that choles-terol-fed apoE knockout mice undergo plaque rupture, but only in the subcla-vian artery. Spontaneous plaque rupture within the coronary arteries has been reported in cholesterol-fed, inbred strains of Watanabe rabbits and with cho-lesterol feeding in mice with genetic deletions of both apoE and the scavenger receptor SR-BI. Interestingly, these animals experience extensive myocardial damage and a high incidence of sudden death.

■ Current Therapeutic Approaches

Lifestyle Modification

- Counseling with regard to dietary modification and performance of regular exer-cise constitute the cornerstone of all approaches to lowering LDL cholesterol.
- Consumption of a balanced diet favoring greater proportions of fruits, vegeta-bles, fiber, seeds, and nuts, with reductions in total and saturated fat and cho-lesterol, should be encouraged. The caloric content of meals should also be addressed. Many people consume infrequent, large-calorie meals. A diet that includes more frequent consumption (every 4 hours) of lower-calorie meals provides a more balanced dietary intake during a 24-hour cycle. The use of plant sterols/stanols as dietary supplements may provide additional assistance in lowering cholesterol.
- Regular exercise should be encouraged for all. The intensity of exercise required is often overestimated by people, who lack motivation. Daily exercise, in the form of brisk walking, swimming, jogging, or cycling, for a duration of 30 min-utes in order to build up a sweat and raise the heart rate is recommended. This is a level of activity that most people should be able to achieve.
- These measures will typically result in reductions in weight and waist circum-ference, with associated reductions in LDL cholesterol and increases in HDL cholesterol, by up to 10%. More substantial reductions in triglyceride levels may be observed in overweight patients with hypertriglyceridemia at baseline.
- Smoking cessation should be emphasized to reduce cardiovascular risk.

Statins

- Statins inhibit HMGCoA reductase, a pivotal factor involved in the synthesis of cholesterol in the liver. Inhibition triggers upregulation of hepatic expression of the LDL receptor, increasing absorption of LDL cholesterol. This results in enhanced clearance and lower systemic levels of LDL cholesterol.
- Dose-dependent reductions in LDL cholesterol in the order of 20% to 60% are observed, with the more recent generation of agents (atorvastatin, rosuvastatin) demonstrating more lowering of LDL cholesterol. Associated reductions in tri-glyceride by up to 30% are observed with the more potent agents. Agents have variable effects on levels of HDL cholesterol, with elevations of 3% to 15%.

- In addition to effects on lipids, it has been proposed that statins possess pleiotropic properties that may contribute to their benefit. These activities are independent of their ability to lower LDL cholesterol and appear to result primarily from inhibition of protein isoprenylation. This has been demonstrated to be associated with anti-inflammatory, antioxidant, and antithrombotic effects in cellular studies, although typically with concentrations much higher than achieved in humans. The potential early benefit of statins in acute coronary syndromes and the relationship of benefit to reductions in inflammatory biomarkers suggest that nonlipid-lowering effects do contribute to reductions in event rates.

- Statins have been the most investigated class of therapeutic agents. Accordingly, substantial information has been collected with regard to their safety. Adverse reactions are encountered much less frequently than with earlier generations of lipid-lowering therapies. Although myalgia is frequently encountered, the incidence of significant elevation of creatine kinase and myopathy is uncommon. Furthermore, the incidence of rhabdomyolosis is rare and often encountered in the setting of an additional risk factor (elderly, concomitant illness, polypharmacy, excess alcohol use). Genomewide association scans have recently identified a polymorphism on chromosome 12 associated with hepatic uptake of statins and subsequent incidence of myopathy. Elevation of liver transaminases are reversible and not associated with demonstrable hepatic pathology. The incidence of hepatic injury as result of statin use is rare. Adverse reactions are more common in patients cotreated with an agent that interacts with cytochrome P450 3A4 metabolism (cyclosporine, fibrates) and are not encountered with the use of pravastatin and fluvastatin, which are metabolized by other mechanisms. Myalgia and transaminase elevation are more typically observed at higher doses. Some patients require dose reduction or use of an alternative agent. Supplementation with coenzyme Q has been proposed as a means to reduce myalgic symptoms, although its use has not been extensively evaluated in clinical trials.

■ Fibric Acid Derivatives

- Fibric acid derivatives act as relatively weak agonists of the nuclear hormone receptor, peroxisome proliferator-activated receptor (PPAR-α), which is involved in regulation of HDL synthesis, reverse cholesterol transport, lipase activity, and inflammatory cascades. As a result, fibrates have more notable effects on triglyceride and HDL cholesterol levels. Clinical studies have demonstrated that fibrates have a beneficial effect on event rates in both primary and secondary prevention and in slow angiographic disease progression in diabetics. Although not typically used for isolated hypercholesterolemia, they may be used in combination with LDL-lowering agents in the setting of combined dyslipidemia or in patients with established coronary heart disease.

■ Cholesterol Absorption Inhibitors

■ Bile acid sequestrants bind to dietary cholesterol and therefore reduce its intestinal absorption. At maximally tolerated doses of 24 to 30 g/day, modest reductions in LDL cholesterol of up to 25% are observed. As a result, these agents are typically used in the management of mild hypercholesterolemia or in combination with other agents. High doses are not frequently achieved, due to intestinal side effects. Effects on bioavailability of other pharmacological therapies (anticoagulants) are variable and require monitoring.

■ Recently, intestinal absorption inhibitors, which act directly at the level of the brush border, have emerged. Ezetimibe has been demonstrated to have a modest effect in lowering LDL cholesterol as monotherapy and provides incremental lowering in combination with statins. While ezetimibe monotherapy does not lower CRP levels, when it is used in combination with statins, CRP levels are reduced to a greater degree than observed with statins alone. These agents appear to be well tolerated and have been proposed by some investigators to be useful for the patient who has not achieved his or her goal despite maximal statin therapy or who cannot tolerate higher statin doses. The recent demonstration that the combination of simvastatin and ezetimibe did not slow progression of carotid intimal-medial thickness compared with simvastatin alone emphasizes the need to further evaluate the effect of this agent on clinical outcomes. A large clinical outcome trial assessing the impact of the combination of statin and ezetimibe is in progress.

■ Nicotinic Acid

■ Nicotinic acid has modest effects in lowering LDL cholesterol, lipoprotein(a), and triglyceride levels, in addition to a significant elevation of HDL cholesterol by up to 35%. This degree of lipid modification is typically observed at higher doses (2 g/day).

■ Early evidence of clinical benefit was observed in the Coronary Drug Project, in which use of niacin reduced the incidence of nonfatal myocardial infarction and long-term mortality in patients with established coronary heart disease. This is supported by reports that niacin slowed progression of carotid intimal-medial thickness and promoted angiographic regression in combination with statin therapy in patients with established heart disease.

■ Nicotinic acid is often used as supplementary therapy for patients with hypercholesterolemia or mixed forms of dyslipidemia, particularly those characterized by low levels of HDL cholesterol.

■ It is often difficult to get patients to achieve effective doses, due to intolerance, particularly flushing. Numerous measures have been attempted, with variable success, to reduce cutaneous flushing. Conservative measures, such as taking medication in the evening and refraining from consumption of caffeine and alcohol, are worthwhile in some patients. Pretreatment with aspirin is recommended to reduce flushing. Patients must be counseled that flushing is common and that titration of therapy will be slow in order to achieve effective doses that are associated with clinical benefit. Extended-release forms of niacin have been reported to reduce, but not eliminate, the incidence of flushing. The recent discovery that flushing results from stimulation of epidermal prostanoid receptors led to the formation of chemical inhibitors that can be administered in combination with niacin. The efficacy of this approach is currently being evaluated in large clinical trials. It is unknown whether prostanoid receptor inhibition has any adverse reactions.

- Additional adverse effects include elevations of liver transaminases and uric acid, kidney and gall stones, and impaired glucose control. As a result, caution should be used with regard to the administration of niacin to patients with gout or diabetes.

■ Partial Ileal Bypass Surgery

- The role of enterohepatic recycling of cholesterol via absorption in the distal small intestine provides the rationale for bypass of the distal ileum as a method to lower cholesterol in patients refractory to dietary and pharmacologic intervention.
- The Program on the Surgical Control of the Hyperlipidemias (POSCH) evaluated the impact of partial ileal bypass surgery in 838 survivors of myocardial infarction, who were followed for 10 years. A 38% reduction in LDL cholesterol was associated with a 35% reduction in the combination of coronary death and myocardial infarction. Less disease progression was observed in these patients on serial angiographic follow-up. Ongoing follow-up for 5 years following completion of the study revealed persistent clinical benefit and reductions in total mortality.
- Adverse effects of ileal bypass surgery include diarrhea, kidney and gallbladder stones, and intestinal obstruction. Most clinical experience with this surgical technique preceded the availability of statins, and as a result it is currently reserved as a therapeutic option for the drug-resistant patient.

■ Primary Prevention Studies of Cholesterol Lowering

- The West of Scotland Coronary Prevention Study (WOSCOPS) evaluated the effect of pravastatin 40 mg on hypercholesterolemic (LDL cholesterol 174–232 mg/dL) men aged 45 to 64 years. A reduction in LDL cholesterol of 26% was associated with a 31% reduction in nonfatal myocardial infarction, a 32% reduction in cardiovascular death, and a 37% reduction in coronary revascularization. The absolute reduction in cardiovascular event rates was in the order of 3%, suggesting that approximately 33 patients would need to be treated to prevent an event. The clinical benefit was apparent after 6 months of treatment. Long-term follow-up of patients revealed that the clinical benefit persisted in the pravastatin-treated group.

- The Air Force/Texas Coronary Atherosclerosis Prevention Study (AFCAPS/TexCAPS) evaluated the effect of lovastatin 20 to 40 mg in 6605 patients without established coronary heart disease and lower levels of LDL cholesterol (average 150 mg/dL). Lowering LDL cholesterol by 25% was associated with a 37% reduction in acute major coronary events, a 40% reduction in myocardial infarction, and a 33% reduction in coronary revascularization after 5 years of follow-up. The 2% absolute reduction in events suggested 50 patients required treatment to prevent an event. Subsequent analysis revealed that lovastatin lowered CRP levels independently of their effect on LDL cholesterol. An elevated baseline CRP level predicted the likelihood that lovastatin would result in clinical benefit.

- The Anglo-Scandinavian Cardiac Outcomes Trial (ASCOT) enrolled 19,342 hypertensive patients with additional cardiovascular risk factors and included both antihypertensive and lipid-lowering arms. Participating in the lipid-lowering arm were 10,305 patients with a total cholesterol <251 mg/dL (6.5 mmol/L); they received atorvastatin 10 mg or placebo. The lipid-lowering arm was stopped early after 3.3 years due to a significant reduction in the combination of nonfatal myocardial infarction and fatal coronary heart disease by 36% with atorvastatin, a benefit that became apparent within the first year of treatment.

- The Justification for the Use of Statins in Primary Prevention: An Intervention Trial Evaluating Rosuvastatin (JUPITER) is a study aimed to test the hypothesis that statin administration would be associated with a clinical benefit in low-risk patients who are not typically considered eligible for lipid-lowering therapy. Patients with a low Framingham risk (10-year risk <10%), LDL cholesterol <130 mg/dL, but a CRP >2 mg/L were treated with rosuvastatin 20 mg or placebo. The study was stopped early due to significant clinical benefit in the rosuvastatin-treated subjects. A 44% reduction in cardiovascular events and a 20% reduction in mortality were observed. This is the first large-scale demonstration of mortality benefit in a primary prevention study. The study highlighted the safety of rosuvastatin in a large cohort of patients and confirms the efficacy of statins in both females and the elderly, groups who have traditionally been underrepresented in primary prevention trials of statin therapy. This extends the benefit of statin therapy to much lower-risk patients than previously demonstrated and highlights the potential of treating patients with evidence of systemic inflammation. Subsequent analyses revealed that subjects achieving the lowest levels of both LDL cholesterol and CRP had the lowest event rates. In addition, venous thromboembolic events were reduced, extending the benefit of statin therapy in this population beyond the arterial tree. (See Table 8-1.)

Table 8-1: Summary of Statin Trials in the Primary Prevention Setting

Trial	Setting	Comparison	Effect on clinical events	Comments
WOSCOPS	Elevated LDL	Pravastatin/ placebo	Decreased myocardial infarction (MI), cardiovascular death, revascularization	Persistent benefit at long-term follow-up
AFCAPS/ TexCAPS	Elevated LDL	Lovastatin/ placebo	Decreased major adverse cardiovascular events (MACE) and revascularization	Low CRP at follow-up predicted greater benefit
ASCOT	Hypertension plus risk factors	Atorvastatin/ placebo	Decreased MACE	
JUPITER	Low LDL with elevated CRP	Rosuvastatin/ placebo	Decreased MACE and mortality	Benefit in patients with evidence of inflammation; mortality reduction in primary prevention; benefits in females and elderly; good safety profile

■ Secondary Prevention Studies of Cholesterol Lowering

■ Patients with established atherosclerotic cardiovascular disease have a high risk of recurrent events. Accordingly, this patient cohort requires the most intensive risk factor modification. Increasing evidence has also highlighted patients with either type 2 diabetes mellitus or multiple risk factors (10-year Framingham risk >20%) as coronary risk equivalents. As a result, these groups also require intensive risk modification, even in the absence of established atherosclerotic disease.

■ The Scandinavian Simvastatin Survival Study (4S) assessed the impact of simvastatin 20 to 40 mg in 4444 patients with established coronary heart disease and total cholesterol 212 to 309 mg/dL (5.5–8.0 mmol/L). After 5.4 years of follow-up, a 35% reduction in LDL cholesterol was associated with a 30% reduction in total mortality, a 34% reduction in cardiovascular events, a 37% reduction in coronary revascularization, and a 28% reduction in stroke. Approximately 30 patients needed to be treated to prevent one event. The greatest impact was observed in patients with low levels of HDL cholesterol and hypertriglyceridemia at baseline. Long-term follow-up of patients revealed persistent clinical benefit for patients randomized to the simvastatin group.

- The Long-Term Intervention with Pravastatin in Ischaemic Disease (LIPID) study evaluated the efficacy of pravastatin in 9014 patients with a recent acute coronary event and total cholesterol 155 to 270 mg/dL (4–7 mmol/L). The study was stopped early after 5 years of follow-up due to significant reductions in mortality, myocardial infarction, stroke, and need for bypass surgery.

- The Cholesterol and Recurrent Events (CARE) study evaluated the impact of pravastatin 40 mg in patients with a previous myocardial infarction but not markedly elevated levels of LDL cholesterol (average 139 mg/dL at baseline). After 5 years of follow-up pravastatin therapy was associated with significant reductions in the combination of coronary death or myocardial infarction by 24%, coronary revascularization by 23% to 26% or stroke by 31%. Thirty-three patients needed treatment to prevent one event during the course of the study. Interestingly and in contrast to the other studies, the benefit was observed only in patients with baseline LDL cholesterol levels greater than 125 mg/dL, and it demonstrated little relationship with the degree of LDL cholesterol lowering.

- The Heart Protection Study (HPS) evaluated simvastatin 40 mg in 20,536 high-risk patients with either established cardiovascular disease, diabetes, or treated hypertension across a broad range of LDL cholesterol levels. After 5.5 years of follow-up, simvastatin was associated with reductions in total mortality by 13%, cardiovascular events by 24%, and stroke by 25%. A similar percentage reduction in events was observed across all tertiles of baseline LDL cholesterol, suggesting that the benefit of simvastatin extended to much lower levels than previously observed.

- The Atorvastatin Versus Revascularization Treatment (AVERT) study compared aggressive lipid lowering with atorvastatin 80 mg and angioplasty in 341 patients with established coronary heart disease with stenoses of 1 or 2 vessels and LDL cholesterol >115 mg/dL (3.0 mmol/L). Lower levels of LDL cholesterol in the atorvastatin group (77 versus 119 mg/dL) were associated with a lower rate of cardiovascular end points, although this failed to meet statistical significance. Rates of bypass surgery and hospitalization for angina were lower in the atorvastatin-treated patients.

- The Collaborative Atorvastatin Diabetes Study (CARDS) evaluated the impact of atorvastatin 10 mg in 2838 diabetic patients with an additional risk factor, no known cardiovascular disease, and an LDL cholesterol <160 mg/dL. The study was stopped prematurely after 3.9 years due to a 37% reduction in cardiovascular events with atorvastatin.

- The Atorvastatin Study for Prevention of Coronary Heart Disease Endpoints in Non-Insulin-Dependent Diabetes Mellitus (ASPEN) evaluated the impact of atorvastatin 10 mg in 2410 diabetic patients either with LDL cholesterol <160 mg/dL (4.1 mmol/L) without known coronary disease or with LDL cholesterol <140 mg/dL (3.6 mmol/L) with known coronary disease.

No significant reduction in cardiovascular events was observed in any subgroup, although it was noted that additional lipid-lowering therapy was initiated more often in placebo patients and that the dropout rate in the study was high.

- A subsequent meta-analysis of more than 90,000 patients enrolled in 14 trials of statin therapy revealed that each 40 mg/dL (1 mmol/L) reduction in LDL cholesterol was associated with approximately a 20% reduction in vascular events during 5 years of follow-up. No adverse effect on cancer rates was demonstrated in statin-treated patients. A 21% reduction in events was more recently observed in the 18,686 diabetic patients.

- The benefit of lipid lowering in patients with regard to stroke has been a subject of considerable debate. The differential profile of risk factors in stroke, as compared with myocardial infarction, suggested that lowering cholesterol may be less important. In support, early studies prior to the use of statins demonstrated that lipid lowering with fibrates, bile acid sequestrants, or diet did not reduce stroke rates. Use of statins, in trials of secondary but not primary prevention demonstrates a beneficial impact on stroke rates. The Stroke Prevention by Aggressive Reduction in Cholesterol Levels (SPARCL) study directly compared atorvastatin 80 mg and placebo in 4731 patients with a stroke or transient ischemic attack in the preceding 6 months, no coronary heart disease, and LDL cholesterol 100 to 190 mg/dL (2.6–4.9 mmol/L). After 4.9 years of follow-up, atorvastatin use was associated with a 16% reduction in stroke and a 26% reduction in cardiovascular events. The reduction in ischemic stroke was partially offset by a minor increase in hemorrhagic events.

- The decision to implement lipid-lowering therapy in elderly patients has received considerable attention. Elderly patients were either not enrolled or underrepresented in the large statin clinical trials. However, there is no convincing evidence from subgroup analysis to suggest that a similar clinical benefit is not observed in elderly patients. The heightened cardiovascular risk in these patients suggests that they may stand to achieve significant clinical benefit from use of therapies. However, the benefits must be considered in the setting of expectations of life span and potential for adverse drug effects, particularly in the patient who is prescribed multiple medications for other medical problems. The Prospective Study of Pravastatin in the Elderly at Risk (PROSPER) compared pravastatin 40 mg and placebo in 8804 patients, aged 70 to 82, with established vascular disease or risk factors. Lowering LDL cholesterol by 34% with pravastatin was associated with a 15% reduction in the combination of coronary death, nonfatal myocardial infarction, and stroke. Although an increase in the rate of cancer was observed, this was not confirmed by subsequent meta-analyses of statin trials. (See Table 8-2.)

Table 8-2: Summary of Statin Trials in the Secondary Prevention and High-Risk Setting

Trial	Setting	Comparison	Effect on clinical events	Comments
4S	Myocardial infarction and elevated LDL	Simvastatin/ placebo	Decreased mortality and MACE	First large-scale of benefit of statin therapy in secondary prevention
LIPID	CHD and elevated LDL	Pravastatin/ placebo	Decreased MACE	
CARE	CHD and lower LDL levels	Pravastatin/ placebo	Decreased MACE	Benefit only in those with baseline LDL >125 mg/dL
HPS	CHD or high risk	Simvastatin/ placebo	Decreased MACE	Benefit regardless of baseline LDL level
AVERT	Stable CHD	Atorvastatin/ placebo	Decreased bypass and hospitalization for angina	
CARDS	Diabetes	Atorvastatin/ placebo	Decrease MACE	
ASPEN	Diabetes	Atorvastatin/ placebo	No benefit	Significant additional therapy in placebo group
SPARCL	Stroke or transient ischemic attack	Atorvastatin/ placebo	Decreased stroke and MACE	
PROSPER	Elderly	Pravastatin/ placebo	Decreased MACE	First prospective benefit in older patients

■ Intensive Cholesterol Lowering

■ The Treating to New Targets (TNT) study compared atorvastatin at low [10 mg, LDL cholesterol goal 100 mg/dL (2.6 mmol/L)] and high [80 mg, LDL cholesterol goal 75 mg/dL (1.9 mmol/L)] doses in 10,001 patients with stable coronary heart disease and baseline LDL cholesterol 130 to 250 mg/dL (3.4–6.5 mmol/L). Use of high-dose atorvastatin was associated with a significant reduction in the primary end point, the combination of death from coronary heart disease, nonfatal myocardial infarction, and resuscitation from cardiac arrest or stroke. High-dose therapy was associated with a greater rate of liver enzyme elevation, but no excess in muscle-related events.

- The Incremental Decrease in End Points Through Aggressive Lipid Lowering (IDEAL) study was an open-labeled comparison of intensive (atorvastatin 80 mg) and standard (simvastatin 20–40 mg) lipid-lowering strategies in 8888 patients with a previous myocardial infarction. Despite lower levels of LDL cholesterol [81 versus 104 mg/dL (2.7 versus 2.1 mmol/L)], the reduction in the primary end point (coronary death, hospitalization for myocardial infarction or cardiac arrest) by 11% just failed to meet statistical significance. Significant reductions in nonfatal myocardial infarction by 17% and coronary revascularization by 23% were observed in the intensive group. More patients in the intensive group stopped therapy due to myalgia and liver enzyme abnormalities.

■ Treatment of the Acute Patient

- The separation of event curves in secondary prevention trials of statin therapy typically occurs after 6 months. However, it has been reported that the anti-inflammatory and antithrombotic activities, in addition to effects on the endothelium described with statins, may translate into an early clinical benefit when administered to patients with acute coronary syndromes.

- The Fluvastatin On Risk Diminishment after Acute myocardial infarction (FLORIDA) study compared fluvastatin 80 mg and placebo in 540 patients with an acute myocardial infarction and total cholesterol <251 mg/dL (6.5 mmol/L). No reduction in cardiovascular end points or ambulatory ischemia was observed after 12 months, although many patients had LDL cholesterol levels that remained above treatment goals.

- The Myocardial Ischemia Reduction with Aggressive Cholesterol Lowering (MIRACL) study compared atorvastatin 80 mg and placebo in 3086 patients 24 to 86 hours after admission for unstable angina or non–Q-wave myocardial infarction. A significant reduction in the composite end point of nonfatal myocardial infarction, resuscitated cardiac arrest, or hospitalization for symptomatic ischemia was observed in atorvastatin-treated patients after 16 weeks.

- The Pravastatin or Atorvastatin Evaluation and Infection Therapy-Thrombolysis in Myocardial Infarction 22 (PROVE IT-TIMI 22) study compared moderate (pravastatin 40 mg) and intensive (atorvastatin 80 mg) lipid-lowering strategies in 4162 patients with an acute coronary syndrome in the preceding 10 days and total cholesterol <240 mg/dL (6.21 mmol/L) with no therapy or <200 mg/dL (5.18 mmol/L). After 24 months of treatment, a lower LDL cholesterol in the intensive treatment group [62 versus 96 mg/dL (1.60 versus 2.46 mmol/L)] was associated with a 16% reduction in the combination of total mortality, myocardial infarction, hospitalization for unstable angina, coronary revascularization, and stroke. The clinical benefit of atorvastatin became apparent after 30 days of treatment. Patients who achieved the greatest lowering of both LDL cholesterol and CRP demonstrated the lowest clinical event rates.

■ The Z phase of A-to-Z compared an aggressive statin strategy (simvastatin 40 mg for one month, followed by 80 mg thereafter) and a delayed conservative statin strategy (placebo for 4 months, followed by simvastatin 20 mg thereafter) in 4497 patients with an acute coronary syndrome and total cholesterol <250 mg/dL (6.48 mmol/L). The 11% reduction in cardiovascular death, myocardial infarction, recurrent acute coronary syndrome, and stroke with the aggressive strategy did not meet statistical significance. In fact, the reduction in the primary end point was observed in the aggressive arm only after 4 months. In addition to the lack of efficacy, a greater rate of substantial creatine kinase elevations was observed in the aggressively treated patients. (See Table 8-3.)

Table 8-3: Summary of Statin Trials of Acute Ischemic Syndromes and Assessing Intensive Lipid Lowering

Trial	Setting	Comparison	Effect on clinical events	Comments
FLORIDA	Postmyocardial infarction	Fluvastatin 80 mg/placebo	No benefit	Small study
MIRACL	Postacute coronary syndrome	Atorvastatin 80 mg/placebo	Decreased MACE	First demonstration of early statin benefit
PROVE IT	Postacute coronary syndrome	Atorvastatin 80 mg/pravastatin 40 mg	Decreased MACE	Benefit of early intensive statin therapy; lowering CRP predicted benefit independently of LDL
A-to-Z	Postacute coronary syndrome	Simvastatin 40–80 mg/placebo to simvastatin 20 mg	No significant benefit	
TNT	Stable CHD	Atorvastatin 80 mg/10 mg	Decreased MACE	
IDEAL	Previous myocardial infarction	Atorvastatin 80 mg/simvastatin 20–40 mg	No significant benefit	

■ When to Intervene

- ■ Increasing evidence that endothelial dysfunction and subclinical atherosclerosis are present in teenagers and young adults supports the need for regular assessment of cardiovascular risk from an early point in life. This is particularly the case for subjects with a family history of premature cardiovascular disease.

- ■ It is currently recommended that all individuals undergo evaluation of a standard lipid profile prior to the age of 30, largely to exclude genetic forms of dyslipidemia.

- ■ All patients with established atherosclerotic cardiovascular disease or those who are determined to be coronary risk equivalents (10-year Framingham risk >20%) should undergo lipid lowering to achieve an LDL cholesterol <100 mg/dL (2.6 mmol/L) with lifestyle modification and pharmacological therapy. An optional treatment goal of 70 mg/dL (1.8 mmol/L) can be considered for patients at very high risk. The overwhelming benefit of statin therapy in secondary prevention, at all levels of LDL cholesterol, suggests that all patients with established coronary heart disease should be treated. There is no evidence to suggest that therapy should be delayed in these patients.

- ■ The decision to commence therapy for primary prevention is made on the basis of the combination of the LDL cholesterol level and cardiovascular risk. An adequate trial (6–8 weeks) of lifestyle modification with diet and exercise should be instituted as the first line of intervention in all patients. If LDL cholesterol levels are >190 mg/dL (4.9 mmol/L) after this trial, pharmacological therapy should be commenced at all levels of cardiovascular risk. In patients with multiple risk factors but low Framingham risk (<10%), therapy should be initiated at LDL cholesterol levels >160 mg/dL (4.1 mmol/L). In the setting of intermediate Framingham risk (10–20%), treatment should be commenced at LDL cholesterol levels >130 mg/dL (3.4 mmol/L).

- ■ Using lifestyle modification and pharmacological therapy if required, the goal should be to lower LDL cholesterol <160 mg/dL in patients with fewer than two cardiovascular risk factors. Defining treatment targets that are 30 mg/dL less than the threshold for initiation of therapy in the presence of multiple risk factors, a goal of 130 mg/dL or 100 mg/dL should be targeted in patients at low and intermediate Framingham risks, respectively.

- ■ If LDL cholesterol levels are acceptable and cardiovascular risk is low, lipids should be monitored every 5 years. Lipid monitoring should be performed more routinely if LDL cholesterol levels are borderline. All patients should be counseled on diet and exercise, regardless of their risk.

- ■ Once initiated, pharmacological management of dyslipidemia involves the need for lifelong use of therapies. Compliance with lipid-lowering therapy is challenging, with as many as 30% of patients stopping treatment within the first year. This is likely due to a combination of the need for chronic therapy, cost, and side effects, such as myalgia. Patients must be counseled regarding the requirement for long-term modification of risk factors. This will have the greatest impact in preventing morbidity and mortality due to cardiovascular disease.

- As the duration of exposure to lipid-modifying therapy continues to increase in individual patients, the long-term sequelae of treatment continue to be defined. Earlier concerns regarding an elevated risk of cancer with either high-dose statin therapy or low LDL cholesterol levels has not been confirmed by large meta-analyses. Similarly, although it has been proposed that long-term statin use may have a beneficial effect on bone density and cognitive function, this has not been established with objective evidence in large cohorts.

■ Combination Therapy

- Although the combination of lifestyle measures and pharmacological mono-therapy can effectively lower LDL cholesterol to target levels, the levels will be suboptimally controlled in many patients. The use of therapies in combination can be an effective strategy to achieve patients' LDL cholesterol goals.
- Statins have been commonly used in combination with all other classes of lipid-lowering therapies to effectively lower levels of LDL cholesterol and triglycerides.
- The use of combination regimens has raised concern regarding a potential increase in adverse events. In particular, the use of fibrates in combination with statins has been reported to be associated with greater rates of myopathy. This was more prevalent in the setting of cerivastatin, which, around 2001, was subsequently been removed from the market due to an excess rate of rhabdomyolysis, particularly in combination with fibrates. Since that time, statins have been effectively used in combination with fibrates and niacin safely. Patients requiring combination therapy require more vigilant monitoring for the incidence of hepatic and muscular events.

■ Management of the Refractory Patient with Familial Hypercholesterolemia

- Patients with familial hypercholesterolemia typically have severe elevations of LDL cholesterol that require the use of combination therapy. In some of these patients, LDL cholesterol levels remain very high despite use of high doses of agents. Given the high risk of premature cardiovascular disease, consideration is given in these patients to use of additional interventions in order to lower LDL cholesterol.
- LDL apheresis involves the extracorporeal removal of LDL cholesterol by plasma exchange or affinity chromatography. Such techniques can potentially remove all apoB-containing particles (lowering LDL cholesterol levels greater

than 50%) and have been reported to render LDL less susceptible to oxidation. When performed one to two times per week, LDL cholesterol levels can be lowered in previously refractory patients. A recent clinical trial that employed intravascular ultrasound has confirmed early anecdotal reports that apheresis can have a beneficial impact on atherosclerosis disease progression. The need for regular procedures, cost, and the limited number of centers with technical expertise restrict the availability of this approach.

- Although partial ileal bypass surgery has not been directly evaluated in clinical trials of drug refractory patients, it provides an additional option with some evidence of clinical efficacy.
- Liver transplantation has been performed in a small number of patients, in order to regenerate the supply of LDL receptor. Portacaval shunting has also been employed in isolated cases, resulting in reduction in generation of LDL particles, although the direct mechanism responsible for this remains to be defined.
- Genetic replacement therapy provides a potential alternative strategy for future consideration. Expression of the VLDL or LDL receptor has been performed in small numbers of patients with dramatic and persistent reduction in levels of LDL cholesterol. The long-term safety and implications of gene therapy remain to be determined.

■ Emerging Therapies

- Antisense therapy directed against the messenger RNA for apoB has been employed in animal models with beneficial effects on levels of atherogenic lipoproteins and atherosclerosis. Preliminary studies in small cohorts of subjects with familial hypercholesterolemia demonstrate significant reductions in apoB and LDL cholesterol with therapy that could potentially be administered as a subcutaneous injection given every 2 to 3 months. The effect of this approach in a broader range of patients has yet to be evaluated in clinical trials.
- Genetic mutations of protease proprotein convertase subtilisin/kexin type 9 (PCSK9) have been implicated in familial forms of hypercholesterolemia. PCSK9 has been identified to play a counterregulatory role in control of cellular cholesterol homeostasis. In the setting of cholesterol depletion, activation of the sterol regulatory element-binding protein (SREBP) leads to increased surface expression of the LDL receptor, favoring cholesterol influx. At the same time, PCSK9 is upregulated and thought to play a role in receptor degradation, thus preventing excess cholesterol influx. It is therefore of interest that polymorphisms of PCSK9 in humans and genetic deletion of PCSK9 in mice are associated with low levels of LDL cholesterol. As a result, considerable interest has focused on the development of PCSK9 inhibitors as adjunct therapy to statins.

▪ Squalene synthase inhibitors intervene at a more distal point in the cholesterol synthetic pathway than statins. The theoretical advantage is their ability to potentially avoid the ubiquinone pathway, proposed to be involved in muscle-related events. Inhibitors with relatively modest effects on LDL cholesterol are in clinical development, which may also be used in combination with lower doses of statins. It remains to be determined whether potential pleiotropic effects observed with statins are lost with this therapeutic approach.

▪ Summary

▪ LDL cholesterol plays a pivotal role in the formation and clinical expression of atherosclerotic cardiovascular disease.
▪ LDL cholesterol should be evaluated in early adulthood to screen for familial dyslipidemias.
▪ Lowering LDL cholesterol by lifestyle measures and pharmacologic therapies represents the cornerstone of approaches to cardiovascular prevention.
▪ The degree of LDL cholesterol lowering required depends on the overall risk profile of the patient.
▪ Increasing evidence suggests that lipid lowering should be commenced early and in an intensive manner in the highest-risk patients.

▪ Suggested Reading

Aikawa M, Rabkin E, Okada Y, et al. Lipid lowering by diet reduces matrix metalloproteinase activity and increases collagen content of rabbit atheroma. A potential mechanism of lesion stabilization. *Circulation*. 1998;97:2433–2444.

Amarenco P, Bogousslavsky J, Callahan A, 3rd, et al. High-dose atorvastatin after stroke or transient ischemic attack. *N Engl J Med*. 2006;355:549–559.

Baigent C, Keech A, Kearney PM, et al. Efficacy and safety of cholesterol-lowering treatment: Prospective meta-analysis of data from 90,056 participants in 14 randomised trials of statins. *Lancet*. 2005;366:1267–1278.

Brown WV. Safety of statins. *Curr Opin Lipidol*. 2008;19:558–562.

Buchwald H, Varco RL, Matts JP, et al. Effect of partial ileal bypass surgery on mortality and morbidity from coronary heart disease in patients with hypercholesterolemia. Report of the Program on the Surgical Control of the Hyperlipidemias (POSCH). *N Engl J Med*. 1990;323:946–955.

Cannon CP, Braunwald E, McCabe CH, et al. Intensive versus moderate lipid lowering with statins after acute coronary syndromes. *N Engl J Med*. 2004;350:1495–1504.

Clofibrate and niacin in coronary heart disease. 1975. *JAMA*. 231:360–381.

Colhoun HM, Betteridge DJ, Durrington PN, et al. Primary prevention of cardiovascular disease with atorvastatin in type 2 diabetes in the Collaborative Atorvastatin Diabetes Study (CARDS): Multicentre randomised placebo-controlled trial. *Lancet*. 2004;364:685–696.

Davidson MH. Novel nonstatin strategies to lower low-density lipoprotein cholesterol. *Curr Atheroscler Rep*. 2009;11:67–70.

de Lemos JA, Blazing MA, Wiviott SD, et al. Early intensive vs a delayed conservative simvastatin strategy in patients with acute coronary syndromes: Phase Z of the A to Z trial. *JAMA*. 2004;292:1307–1316.

Downs JR, Clearfield M, Weis S, et al. Primary prevention of acute coronary events with lovastatin in men and women with average cholesterol levels: Results of AFCAPS/TexCAPS. AirForce/Texas Coronary Atherosclerosis Prevention Study. *JAMA*. 1998;279:1615–1622.

Influence of pravastatin and plasma lipids on clinical events in the West of Scotland Coronary Prevention Study (WOSCOPS). *Circulation*. 1998;97:1440–1445.

Knopp RH, d'Emden M, Smilde JG, Pocock SJ. Efficacy and safety of atorvastatin in the prevention of cardiovascular end points in subjects with type 2 diabetes: The Atorvastatin Study for Prevention of Coronary Heart Disease Endpoints in non-insulin-dependent diabetes mellitus (ASPEN). *Diabetes Care*. 2006;29:1478–1485.

LaRosa JC, Grundy SM, Waters DD, et al. Intensive lipid lowering with atorvastatin in patients with stable coronary disease. *N Engl J Med*. 2005;352:1425–1435.

Liem AH, van Boven AJ, Veeger NJ, et al. Effect of fluvastatin on ischaemia following acute myocardial infarction: A randomized trial. *Eur Heart J*. 2002;23:1931–1937.

The Long-Term Intervention with Pravastatin in Ischaemic Disease (LIPID) Study Group. Prevention of cardiovascular events and death with pravastatin in patients with coronary heart disease and a broad range of initial cholesterol levels. *N Engl J Med*. 1998;339:1349–1357.

MRC/BHF Heart Protection Study of cholesterol lowering with simvastatin in 20,536 high-risk individuals: A randomised placebo-controlled trial. *Lancet*. 2002;360:7–22.

Nissen SE, Nicholls SJ, Sipahi I, et al. Effect of very high-intensity statin therapy on regression of coronary atherosclerosis: The ASTEROID trial. *JAMA*. 2006;295:1556–1565.

Nissen SE, Tuzcu EM, Schoenhagen P, et al. Effect of intensive compared with moderate lipid-lowering therapy on progression of coronary atherosclerosis: A randomized controlled trial. *JAMA*. 2004;291:1071–1080.

Pedersen TR, Faergeman O, Kastelein JJ, et al. High-dose atorvastatin vs usual-dose simvastatin for secondary prevention after myocardial infarction: The IDEAL study: A randomized controlled trial. *JAMA*. 2005;294:2437–2445.

Pitt B, Waters D, Brown WV, et al. Aggressive lipid-lowering therapy compared with angioplasty in stable coronary artery disease. Atorvastatin versus Revascularization Treatment Investigators. *N Engl J Med*. 1999;341:70–76.

Randomised trial of cholesterol lowering in 4444 patients with coronary heart disease: The Scandinavian Simvastatin Survival Study (4S). *Lancet*. 1994;344:1383–1389.

Ridker PM, Danielson E, Fonseca FA, et al. Rosuvastatin to prevent vascular events in men and women with elevated C-reactive protein. *N Engl J Med*. 2008;359:2195–2207.

Sacks FM, Pfeffer MA, Moye LA, et al. The effect of pravastatin on coronary events after myocardial infarction in patients with average cholesterol levels. Cholesterol and Recurrent Events Trial investigators. *N Engl J Med*. 1996;335:1001–1009.

Schwartz GG, Olsson AG, Ezekowitz MD, et al. Effects of atorvastatin on early recurrent ischemic events in acute coronary syndromes: The MIRACL study: A randomized controlled trial. *JAMA*. 2001;285:1711–1718.

Secondary prevention by raising HDL cholesterol and reducing triglycerides in patients with coronary artery disease: The Bezafibrate Infarction Prevention (BIP) study. *Circulation.* 2000;102:21–27.

Seidah NG. PCSK9 as a therapeutic target of dyslipidemia. *Expert Opin Ther Targets.* 2009;13:19–28.

Shepherd J, Blauw GJ, Murphy MB, et al. Pravastatin in elderly individuals at risk of vascular disease (PROSPER): A randomised controlled trial. *Lancet.* 2002;360:1623–1630.

Shepherd J, Cobbe SM, Ford I, et al. Prevention of coronary heart disease with pravastatin in men with hypercholesterolemia. West of Scotland Coronary Prevention Study Group. *N Engl J Med.* 1995;333:1301–1307.

Thompson GR. Recommendations for the use of LDL apheresis. *Atherosclerosis.* 2008;198:247–255.

CHAPTER 9

HDL Cholesterol

■ Background

- The highest-density lipoproteins in the systemic circulation consist of a core of esterified cholesterol and triglyceride, surrounded by surface monolayer of phospholipid and a range of apolipoproteins (A-I, A-II, A-IV, C-I, C-II, C-III, and E).
- The particles are heterogeneous in terms of size, shape, electrophoretic mobility, and composition of protein, cholesterol, triglyceride, and phospholipid.
- Substantial evidence suggests that HDL plays a protective role in vivo.

■ Population Studies

- An early report by Barr and colleagues demonstrated that patients admitted to coronary care units with myocardial infarction had low levels of lipid particles with α mobility, consistent with HDL. Subsequent case control series demonstrated that low HDL cholesterol levels are associated with increased cardiovascular risk.
- Numerous large population studies demonstrated an inverse relationship between systemic levels of HDL cholesterol and the prospective risk of cardiovascular events, independent of levels of LDL cholesterol. HDL cholesterol levels were found to be the strongest biochemical predictor of cardiovascular risk in the Framingham Heart Study.
- Despite the association between low levels of HDL cholesterol and hypertriglyceridemia, the PROCAM (Prospective Cardiovascular Munster) study revealed that a low HDL cholesterol level predicts an increased risk at all triglyceride levels.
- A pooled analysis of four population studies revealed that each 1 mg/dL increase in HDL cholesterol is associated with a 2% to 3% reduction in cardiovascular risk.
- Low HDL cholesterol levels are the most commonly encountered lipid abnormality in patients attending cardiology outpatient clinics and in patients with premature coronary artery disease.
- Low HDL cholesterol levels predict an adverse outcome following percutaneous coronary intervention.

- As a result, HDL cholesterol has become an integral component of risk prediction algorithms. A low level (<40 mg/dL in men and <50 mg/dL in women) counts as a risk factor. The protective role of a level >60 mg/dL allows for one other risk factor to not be counted.

■ Animal Studies

- Badimon and colleagues were the first to report that infusions of HDL retarded lesion formation and promoted regression of established lesions in cholesterol-fed rabbit models of atherosclerosis. Raising HDL cholesterol levels by transgenic expression of human apoA-I reduced lesion size in mouse models of atherosclerosis.
- Promoting HDL activity by transgenic expression of apoA-I or infusion of HDL reduced the inflammatory composition of established atherosclerotic lesions, consistent with plaque stabilization.
- Infusion of HDL attenuated development of restenosis due to neointima formation in stented regions.

■ Role of HDL in Reverse Cholesterol Transport

- The best characterized role of HDL is its role in the facilitation of reverse cholesterol transport. (See Figure 9-1.) HDL has been demonstrated to accept cholesterol effluxed from cells via a number of mechanisms. Simple diffusion of cholesterol from cells to HDL particles follows a concentration gradient. Energy-dependent transfer of cholesterol and phospholipid from cells to HDL occurs via the transmembrane protein, ATP (adenosine triphosphate) binding cassette A-1 (ABCA-1). Discoidal, lipid-deplete HDL particles are the preferred acceptors for interaction with ABCA-1. The scavenger receptor, SR-BI, has been identified to facilitate bidirectional flux of cholesterol between cells and large HDL particles. More recently, ABCG-1 has been identified as a facilitator of cholesterol efflux to large, cholesterol-rich HDL particles.
- On the HDL surface, free cholesterol is esterified by the factor lecithin:cholesterol acyltransferase (LCAT) and stored within the particle core. This tends to maintain a low surface concentration of cholesterol, favoring ongoing movement from cells to HDL.
- Cholesterol is transported to the liver by spherical HDL particles, where it is taken up via an interaction with SR-BI on the liver surface.
- Cholesterol is also transferred to apoB-containing particles, in exchange for triglyceride, in a process facilitated by cholesteryl ester transfer protein (CETP). Although this process enriches potentially atherogenic lipid particles with cholesterol, it also provides an alternative pathway for return of cholesterol to the liver, where it is taken up by the LDL receptor.
- Numerous groups have attempted to characterize the impact of factors on mechanisms of cholesterol efflux and reverse cholesterol transport in cellular

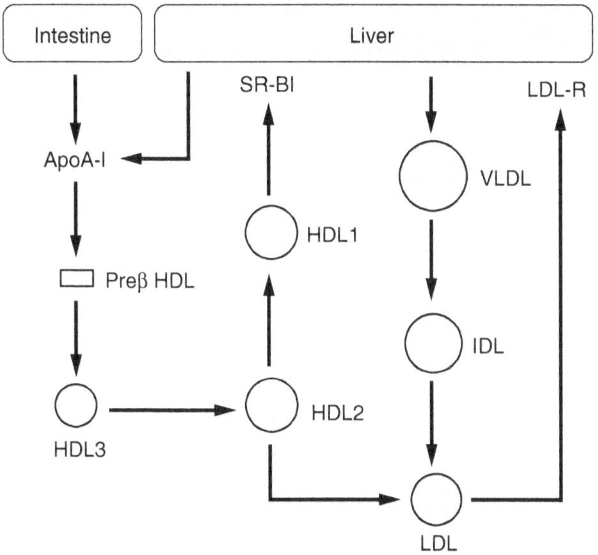

Figure 9-1: Schematic illustration of proposed pathways involved in reverse cholesterol transport. Apolipoprotein A-I (apoA-I) synthesized by the liver and small intestine is rapidly lipidated in the circulation to form discoidal preβ HDL, which acts as the preferred acceptor for efflux via ABCA1. Cholesterol esterification by lecithin:cholesterol acyltransferase results in larger HDL particles that accept cholesterol effluxed via ABCG1 and SR-BI mediated pathways. Cholesterol within HDL is either taken up by the liver via a SR-BI mediated process or is transferred to LDL particles in a process facilitated by cholesteryl ester transfer protein (CETP). Hepatic uptake of cholesterol from LDL via the LDL receptor therefore represents a potential alternative pathway for hepatic uptake in reverse cholesterol transport.

systems and in vivo models. No one single cellular model reliably reflects the totality of efflux mechanisms that have been identified in humans. Measurements of fecal sterol excretion have been employed as a surrogate measure of reverse cholesterol transport. More recently, in vivo models that involve the injection of macrophages containing isotope-labelled cholesterol and the monitoring of the fecal excretion of the radiolabel have been developed. Considerable debate continues to focus on the precision by which these models reflect in vivo processes in humans.

■ **Additional Functional Properties of HDL**

▦ Increasing experimental evidence has demonstrated that HDL possesses functional activities in addition to promoting cholesterol efflux and reverse cholesterol efflux.

▦ A number of antioxidant properties of HDL have been observed. HDL inhibits the formation of lipid hydroperoxides on LDL particles. HDL inhibits generation of superoxide, a pivotal oxidant mediator of vascular disease. Increasing interest has focused on the role of paraoxonase (PON), a factor circulating predominantly on HDL particles that possess antioxidant properties. Genetic manipulation of PON activity is protective in animal models of atherosclerosis. Recent findings that polymorphisms resulting in increased PON activity are associated with reduced markers of systemic oxidative stress, suggesting that antioxidant activity contributes to protection against coronary heart disease.

■ HDLs are reported to possess anti-inflammatory properties, which include their ability to:
  ● inhibit expression of adhesion molecules and chemokines by endothelial cells and subsequent monocyte migration in response to cytokine stimulation,
  ● impair activation and degranulation of leukocytes,
  ● inhibit the inflammatory response following administration of lipopolysaccharide, and
  ● have beneficial effects in the setting of septic shock.

■ HDL enhances the bioavailability of nitric oxide with a beneficial impact on vascular reactivity. This is likely to occur via an SR-BI-mediated mechanism. Infusing HDL in humans improves endothelial-dependent vascular reactivity in subjects with familial hypercholesterolemia and low levels of HDL cholesterol due to heterozygous ABCA-1 deficiency.

■ HDL possesses functional properties that may have a beneficial impact on the prevention of plaque rupture, including their ability to
  ● inhibit endothelial and smooth muscle cell apoptosis, and
  ● inhibit expression of metalloproteinases.

■ HDL has a favorable impact on thrombogenicity by:
  ● inhibiting platelet activation and aggregation,
  ● inhibiting expression of a number of factors involved in activation of the coagulation cascade, and
  ● promoting expression of thrombomodulin and inhibiting PAI-1 (plasminogen activator inhibitor), factors inhibiting thrombosis and promoting fibrinolysis.

■ HDL has also been reported to prevent ischemia-reperfusion injury in organ bath and animal models. This is likely to be derived from a combination of effects on oxidative stress, inflammation, and nitric oxide bioavailability.

■ Dysfunctional HDL

■ Patients are encountered in clinical practice with elevated levels of HDL cholesterol and prevalent coronary heart disease. Although this combination may result from the presence of a large risk factor burden, despite the HDL cholesterol level, it has also been proposed that HDL particles may not be protective in these patients.

- HDL isolated from patients with coronary heart disease despite high HDL cholesterol levels has been demonstrated to promote, rather than inhibit, monocyte migration in response to stimulation with oxidized LDL. This suggests that HDL may be proinflammatory in some subjects.
- A number of groups have suggested that HDL functionality may potentially be modified. The anti-inflammatory activity of HDL is enhanced with statin therapy and following consumption of polyunsaturated fat. In contrast, this activity is impaired following consumption of saturated fat.
- A number of chemical pathways have been implicated in the generation of potentially dysfunctional HDL. Oxidation by either myeloperoxidase, carbamylation, or glycation has been demonstrated to impair HDL functionality in vitro.
- Considerable interest has focused on the development of biomarkers that evaluate HDL functionality both to assess risk and to monitor efficacy of therapies.

■ Current Therapeutic Approaches

- Lifestyle measures—including dietary modification and exercise with weight loss, as well as smoking cessation—are associated with modest elevations of HDL cholesterol by up to 10%. These measures should be initiated as the first line of intervention to elevate HDL cholesterol. Mild consumption of alcohol can elevate HDL cholesterol, although this must be balanced with the effects of alcohol on weight, triglyceride levels, and liver function. (See Table 9-1.)
- Statins raise HDL cholesterol by 3% to 15%, with differences observed among individual agents. The precise mechanism responsible for this elevation remains to be defined, although it is likely to involve an increase in apoA-I production, decrease of its renal excretion, and inhibition of CETP activity. Low baseline levels of HDL cholesterol identified the patients likely to derive the greatest clinical benefit in placebo-controlled trials of statin therapy. Raising HDL cholesterol has been identified as an independent predictor of the benefit of statins on clinical events and plaque progression in clinical trials.
- Fibrates elevate HDL cholesterol by 5% to 20%. Primary mode of action is as a pharmacological agonist of the PPAR-α (peroxisome proliferator-activated) receptor, with beneficial effects on several factors involved in HDL metabolism (apoA-I, apoA-II, ABCA-1, SR-BI, and lipoprotein lipase). In a similar fashion to statins, patients with low levels of HDL cholesterol derived the greatest clinical benefit of fibrate therapy in randomized placebo-controlled trials. Modest elevations of HDL cholesterol independently predicted the clinical benefit of gemfibrozil in studies of primary and secondary prevention. Subsequent studies that employed nuclear magnetic resonance analysis of lipid particle and size revealed that increasing small, but not large, HDL particles predicted the clinical benefit of gemfibrozil.

Table 9-1:   Current and Emerging Approaches to Promote HDL Function

Current approaches:	
Diet and exercise	Elevate HDL cholesterol up to 10%
Statins	Elevate HDL cholesterol 3% to 15% depending on agent
	Mechanism for elevation uncertain
	Contribute to benefit of agents in clinical trials
Fibrates	Elevate HDL cholesterol 5% to 20%
	Activation of PPAR-α increases apoA-I and apoA-II in addition to regulating expression of factors promoting reverse cholesterol transport
Niacin	Elevates HDL cholesterol up to 35%
	Mechanism for elevation uncertain
	Developments to limit flushing may improve tolerance.
Pioglitazone	Elevates HDL cholesterol 10% to 15%
	Contributes to benefit on atheroma progression
Emerging approaches:	
Direct administration	Reconstituted or delipidated HDL
	ApoA-I or mutant forms
	Phospholipid vesicles
	ApoA-I mimetic peptides
Remodeling pathways	Cholesteryl ester transfer protein
	Endothelial lipase
Transcription regulation	PPAR
	Liver X receptors
	ApoA-I production
HDL proteomics	Paraoxonase activity
Dysfunctional HDL	Inhibit oxidative stress and inflammatory pathways

■ Niacin is the most effective HDL cholesterol-raising agent (by up to 35%) currently available in clinical practice. The mechanism underlying elevation of HDL cholesterol remains unclear. Early evidence from the Coronary Drug Project revealed that administration of niacin reduced the incidence of nonfatal myocardial infarction and long-term mortality. When used in combination with statin therapy, niacin promotes angiographic regression and slows progression of carotid intimal-medial thickness in patients with coronary heart disease. Cutaneous flushing and adverse effects on glycemic control, uric acid levels, and liver enzymes have limited its use at effective doses (in the order of 2 g daily). Initiation of low-dose therapy with a slow increased titration, in patients who coadminister low-dose aspirin and avoid caffeine, is recommended to achieve long-term effective doses in patients. Patients must be counseled that flushing is common and can be tolerated in many cases, allowing administration of doses that have favorable effects on lipid profile and clinical outcome. Extended-release forms of niacin are reported to lower the incidence of flushing. More recently, activation of epidermal prostanoid receptors has been identified as the mechanism underlying niacin-induced flushing. Preparations that combine niacin and a prostanoid receptor inhibitor (laropiprant) are currently being investigated in large trials to evaluate their impact on clinical outcome.

■ The PPAR-γ agonist, pioglitazone, raises HDL cholesterol by approximately 15%. Raising HDL cholesterol has been demonstrated to independently predict the ability of pioglitazone to slow progression of carotid intimal-medial thickness in patients with type 2 diabetes.

■ The endocannabinoid receptor antagonist, rimonabant, is currently being investigated for impact on clinical outcome in patients with abdominal obesity. Reductions in abdominal adiposity have been reported to be associated with substantial elevations in HDL cholesterol (by more than 20%), although it remains to be determined whether this will result in clinical benefit.

■ CETP Inhibition

■ CETP facilitates the transfer of esterified cholesterol, in exchange for triglyceride, from HDL to apoB-containing particles.

■ The overall impact of CETP on atherosclerosis remains to be determined. The transfer of esterified cholesterol to LDL particles may potentially increase the atherogenic load on the artery wall. In contrast, hepatic uptake of cholesterol from LDL via the LDL receptor provides an alternative pathway contributing to reverse cholesterol transport.

■ Population studies demonstrate variable associations among subjects with low levels of CETP activity and cardiovascular risk. Although some populations with a high incidence of low CETP activity have a low risk of cardiovascular disease, other populations include subjects with premature atherosclerosis.

Genetic polymorphisms associated with low CETP activity have been demonstrated to be associated with reduced cardiovascular risk in several cohorts.

■ Inhibition of CETP activity using vaccines, oligosense nucleotides, and chemical inhibitors has a beneficial impact on lesion size in rabbit models of atherosclerosis. Unlike rabbits, mice do not express CETP and are therefore not useful animal models to evaluate therapeutic strategies to reduce CETP activity.

■ Administration of oral CETP inhibitors in humans raises HDL cholesterol levels by 30% to 100% and reduces LDL cholesterol by up to 20% on top of statin therapy.

■ Inhibition of CETP generates large, cholesterol-enriched HDL particles. Observations that small, lipid-deplete HDL particles are the preferred acceptor of cholesterol effluxed via the ABCA-1 transporter raised speculation that cholesterol efflux activity may be impaired with CETP inhibition. Blockade of cholesterol transfer to LDL particles may have a detrimental impact on reverse cholesterol transport. Accordingly, it has been proposed that CETP inhibition may have an adverse influence on removal of cholesterol from the artery wall and thus promote, rather than inhibit, atherosclerosis formation and propagation.

■ Early clinical studies in humans demonstrated that administration of CETP inhibitors did not impair the cholesterol efflux activity of isolated HDL. Similarly, fecal sterol excretion, a surrogate marker of reverse cholesterol transport, is not reduced following administration of CETP inhibitors.

■ Torcetrapib is the first CETP inhibitor to reach an advanced stage of clinical development. A large clinical event trial of torcetrapib, with background atorvastatin therapy, was stopped early due to an excess rate of mortality with the CETP inhibitor. Two clinical trials that evaluated the impact of torcetrapib on changes in carotid intimal-medial thickness in cohorts with familial hypercholesterolemia and mixed dyslipidemia failed to show a beneficial impact on disease progression, compared with placebo, in atorvastatin-treated subjects. In an additional study, torcetrapib failed to slow progression of coronary atherosclerosis.

■ The lack of efficacy of torcetrapib has fueled speculation regarding the impact of CETP inhibition on HDL functionality. An inverse relationship between changes in levels of HDL cholesterol and disease progression suggests that the particles retain functionality in terms of their ability to mobilize lipids. Recent observations that torcetrapib activates the renin-angiotensin-aldosterone axis provides a mechanism for off-target toxicity of torcetrapib that may mitigate any potential benefit of raising HDL cholesterol.

■ Additional CETP inhibitors that lack such off-target toxicity are currently in clinical development and may still have a protective effect on cardiovascular disease, although this remains to be established in clinical trials. Two agents, dalcetrapib and anacetrapib, are currently in development. Recent reports suggest that these agents lack renin-angiotensin-aldosterone toxicity. Dalcetrapib has already entered a large-scale morbidity-mortality trial in patients with a recent acute coronary syndrome.

■ Infusional HDL Therapy

- Preclinical studies report that intravenous infusions of apoA-I and reconstituted forms of HDL have a beneficial effect on endothelial function and fecal sterol excretion, a surrogate marker of reverse cholesterol transport.
- An early pilot study demonstrated that five weekly intravenous infusions of reconstituted HDL containing phospholipid and recombinant apoA-I Milano (AIM) promoted rapid regression of coronary atherosclerosis. This supports the concept that HDL is beneficial in humans and supports a large body of evidence that AIM is protective and that lipid-poor forms of HDL are efficient promoters of lipid efflux, promoting disease regression.
- Considerable debate has focused on whether AIM possess superior protective properties compared with wild-type apoA-I. A similar study demonstrated that infusion of HDL particles containing wild-type apoA-I had a beneficial effect on atheroma volume and on changes in plaque echogenicity, suggesting a favorable impact on plaque composition.
- The benefits of infusing lipid-deplete forms of HDL on the artery wall in humans has fueled interest in the potential to selectively delipidate a patient's HDL for subsequent reinfusion. Preliminary imaging studies have demonstrated that this approach can also promote rapid disease regression.
- Interest has also focused on the potential to infuse phospholipid vesicles. Following intravenous infusion, phospholipid rapidly associates with apoA-I, becoming assimilated into HDL, potentially slowing HDL metabolism, and elevating HDL cholesterol levels. Phospholipid vesicles promote efflux and are atheroprotective in animal models. The fatty acid composition of the phospholipid may be important. This is supported by observations that the anti-inflammatory activity of HDL is impaired with saturated-fat-rich meals and enhanced following consumption of polyunsaturated fat.
- The impact of infusional therapy on clinical outcome remains to be tested in prospective clinical trials. It also remains to be determined whether infusional HDL therapy will be used in the acute setting to stabilize disease while chronic oral therapies are commenced.

■ Emerging Therapeutic Strategies

- Development of new therapeutic strategies to promote the biological activity of HDL is of immense interest. A range of agents is currently being investigated, primarily with effects on either altering HDL remodeling or enhancing the bioavailability of apoA-I.
- Endothelial lipase (EL) hydrolyzes HDL phospholipids and generates apoA-I that is renally excreted. EL expression in animals is associated with increased

apoA-I catabolism, decreased HDL cholesterol levels, and lesion formation in animal models of atherosclerosis. The inverse correlation between EL levels and coronary calcification further suggests that inhibiting EL may be beneficial. No EL inhibitor has yet to reach clinical development.

- Given that fibrates are relatively weak PPAR-α agonists, there is considerable interest in the potential efficacy of more potent PPAR-α or dual PPAR-$\alpha/\gamma/\delta$ agonists. The theoretical benefit either of a more pronounced effect on HDL cholesterol and reverse cholesterol transport or of the ability to combine this strategy with improving glycemic control and anti-inflammatory activity provides attractive targets for cardiovascular risk reduction. However, no agent with superior efficacy, without toxicity, has reached an advanced stage of clinical development.

- Association of the liver X receptor (LXR) and retinoid X receptor plays a pivotal role in regulating expression of ABCA-1 and ABCG-1. Activation of LXR has beneficial effects on cholesterol efflux, reverse cholesterol transport, and atherosclerosis in animal models. Early LXR agonists enhance fatty acid and triglyceride production by the liver as a result of upregulation of sterol regulatory element-binding protein (SREBP). Therapeutic efficacy in this class is likely to require more selective targeting of LXR in a way that only modifies macrophages or avoids SREBP.

- Short peptides that share no sequence homology with apoA-I but that form amphipathic helices, like apoA-I, have been reported to have a beneficial impact on cholesterol efflux, inflammation, endothelial function, and atherosclerosis in animal models. Preparation of peptides containing D-type amino acids, which are resistant to degradation by gastric enzymes, provides the opportunity for oral administration. Early studies in humans demonstrate that peptide administration results in the presence of anti-inflammatory HDL. The impact on the vessel wall and cardiovascular risk in humans remain to be determined.

- Strategies that induce apoA-I synthesis may have the greatest therapeutic potential. Chemical compounds that enhance hepatic apoA-I synthesis are in clinical development. ApoA-I is also an attractive target for the use of gene therapy, particularly in patients with familial apoA-I deficiency.

- As the chemical pathways that modify HDL and result in functional impairment continue to be elucidated, a number of potential therapeutic strategies will emerge. The ability to inhibit components of the myeloperoxidase and carbamylation pathways may preserve the functionality of circulating HDL particles.

■ Summary

- A large body of evidence is in favor of a protective role of HDL.
- Measuring HDL cholesterol is an integral component of cardiovascular risk prediction algorithms.
- Modest effects on HDL cholesterol contribute to the clinical benefit of current classes of lipid-modifying therapies.

- Considerable interest has focused on the development of new therapies that substantially raise HDL cholesterol.
- Relative functionality of HDL has become increasingly important in terms of risk prediction and development of new therapies.
- Although there is currently no established treatment target for HDL cholesterol, it would seem appropriate to elevate levels to more than 40 mg/dL in men and 50 mg/dL in women.

■ Suggested Reading

Badimon JJ, Badimon L, Fuster V. Regression of atherosclerotic lesions by high density lipoprotein plasma fraction in the cholesterol-fed rabbit. *J Clin Invest.* 1990;85: 1234–1241.

Barter PJ. CETP and atherosclerosis. *Arterioscler Thromb Vasc Biol.* 2000;20:2029–2031.

Barter PJ. Hugh Sinclair lecture: The regulation and remodelling of HDL by plasma factors. *Atherosclerosis Suppl.* 2002;3:39–47.

Barter PJ, Chapman MJ, Hennekens CH, Rader DJ, Tall AR. Cholesteryl ester transfer protein. A novel target for raising HDL and inhibiting atherosclerosis. *Arterioscler Thromb Vasc Biol.* 2003;23:160–167.

Barter PJ, Nicholls S, Rye KA, Anantharamaiah GM, Navab M, Fogelman AM. Antiinflammatory properties of HDL. *Circ Res.* 2004;95:764–772.

Bots ML, Visseren FL, Evans GW, et al. Torcetrapib and carotid intima-media thickness in mixed dyslipidaemia (RADIANCE 2 study): A randomised, double-blind trial. *Lancet.* 2007;370:153–160.

Fielding CJ, Fielding PE. Molecular physiology of reverse cholesterol transport. *J Lipid Res.* 1995;36:211.

Glomset JA. The plasma lecithins: Cholesterol acyltransferase reaction. *J Lipid Res.* 1968;9:155–167.

Gordon DJ, Rifkind BM. High-density lipoprotein—The clinical implications of recent studies. *N Engl J Med.* 1989;321:1311–1316.

Kastelein JJ, van Leuven SI, Burgess L, et al. Effect of torcetrapib on carotid atherosclerosis in familial hypercholesterolemia. *N Engl J Med.* 2007;356:1620–1630.

Nicholls SJ, Cutri B, Worthley SG, et al. Impact of short-term administration of high-density lipoproteins and atorvastatin on atherosclerosis in rabbits. *Arterioscler Thromb Vasc Biol.* 2005;25:2416–2421.

Nicholls SJ, Nissen SE. New targets of high-density lipoprotein therapy. *Curr Opin Lipidol.* 2007;18:421–426.

Nicholls SJ, Tuzcu EM, Brennan DM, Tardif JC, Nissen SE. Cholesteryl ester transfer protein inhibition, high-density lipoprotein raising, and progression of coronary atherosclerosis: Insights from ILLUSTRATE (Investigation of Lipid Level Management Using Coronary Ultrasound to Assess Reduction of Atherosclerosis by CETP Inhibition and HDL Elevation). *Circulation.* 2008;118:2506–2514.

Nicholls SJ, Tuzcu EM, Sipahi I, et al. Statins, high-density lipoprotein cholesterol, and regression of coronary atherosclerosis. *JAMA.* 2007;297:499–508.

Nicholls SJ, Zheng L, Hazen SL. Formation of dysfunctional high-density lipoprotein by myeloperoxidase. *Trends Cardiovasc Med.* 2005;15:212–219.

Nissen SE, Tardif JC, Nicholls SJ, et al. Effect of torcetrapib on the progression of coronary atherosclerosis. *N Engl J Med*. 2007;356:1304–1316.

Nissen SE, Tsunoda T, Tuzcu EM, et al. Effect of recombinant ApoA-I Milano on coronary atherosclerosis in patients with acute coronary syndromes: A randomized controlled trial. *JAMA*. 2003;290:2292–2300.

Oram JF. HDL apolipoproteins and ABCA1. Partners in the removal of excess cellular cholesterol. *Arterioscler Thromb Vasc Biol*. 2003;23:720–727.

Tardif JC, Gregoire J, L'Allier PL, et al. Effects of reconstituted high-density lipoprotein infusions on coronary atherosclerosis: A randomized controlled trial. *JAMA*. 2007;297:1675–1682.

Wang Z, Nicholls SJ, Rodriguez ER, et al. Protein carbamylation links inflammation, smoking, uremia and atherogenesis. *Nat Med*. 2007;13:1146–1147.

Triglycerides

■ Background

■ Triglycerides come from both exogenous and endogenous sources and are vehicles for energy storage, primarily in adipose tissue.

■ There is increasing evidence that triglycerides contribute to the risk of developing coronary heart disease (CHD).

■ The inverse relationship between triglycerides and HDL cholesterol, along with the association between triglycerides and other metabolic abnormalities, complicates analyses of their contributions to CHD.

■ Triglyceride Metabolism

■ The predominant ingested lipids are triglycerides, which constitute approximately 97% of the dietary lipids.

■ Triglycerides are almost completely absorbed from the gut, whereas cholesterol absorption is less efficient and shows greater individual variation. The absorption of dietary lipids is also important for the uptake of vitamins.

■ Triglycerides consist of a glycerol backbone with three fatty acids esterified to the carbon atoms. Triglycerides are the major energy store in the body, particularly in adipose tissue.

■ Fatty acids derived from triglycerides are released through the action of hormone-sensitive lipase, an enzyme that is active during fasting when insulin levels are low. Free fatty acids (FFAs), which circulate in plasma bound to albumin, can be utilized by the muscles as fuel directly or following partial oxidation in the liver to ketone bodies. Ketone bodies are in turn used as fuel by extrahepatic tissues, including the brain.

■ Triglycerides are highly hydrophobic and insoluble in the aqueous plasma environment. They are solubilized by their incorporation into lipoproteins. The triglyceride content in the triglyceride-rich lipoproteins (TRLs)—chylomicrons and VLDLs—forms a central hydrophobic core, together with cholesterol esters, which is surrounded by free cholesterol, phospholipids, and apolipoproteins.

■ Triglyceride-rich Lipoproteins of Exogenous Origin

■ Ingested triglycerides are hydrolyzed to FFAs and monoacylglycerols, mainly by intestinal pancreatic lipase. Monoacylglycerols, FFAs, free cholesterol, and phospholipids, after emulsification and incorporation by bile acids into micelles, are absorbed by the mucosa cells (enterocytes). Chylomicrons are formed in the enterocytes, carrying the majority of the ingested triglycerides, from monoacylglycerols and re-esterified fatty acids. They are packed together with cholesterol esters, free cholesterol, phospholipids, apoA-I, and the intestine-specific apoB48.

- Chylomicrons are rapidly transported from the enterocytes, via the intestinal lymphatic system to the thoracic duct and into the plasma compartment. Short- and medium-chained fatty acids ($\leq$12 carbon atoms) are secreted directly from the enterocytes into the portal vein and transported to the liver.

■ Triglyceride-rich Lipoproteins of Endogenous Origin

- The endogenous source of triglycerides in plasma is VLDL. This lipoprotein is formed in the liver by the coupling of liver-derived triglycerides and cholesterol to the liver-specific apoB100. Intrahepatic triglyceride lipolysis to fatty acids and to fatty acid flux to the liver from adipose tissue and intestine is an important determinant of hepatic triglyceride synthesis and VLDL secretion. Newly secreted VLDLs are heterogeneous in size and density.

- The microsomal triglyceride transfer protein has an important role in the regulation of VLDL secretion and affects the distribution between large and small VLDL particles. The structure of VLDL is similar to that of chylomicrons. However, VLDLs are smaller and denser, and they contain relatively more cholesterol than chylomicrons.

■ Metabolism of Triglyceride-rich Lipoproteins in Hypertriglyceridemia

- Plasma triglyceride levels are dependent both on the production and on the clearance rate of triglyceride-rich lipoproteins.

- During fasting, there are low levels of chylomicron and their remnants in plasma, and the triglyceride level is accounted for by VLDL and their remnants.

- In contrast, in the postprandial state, chylomicrons and their remnants carry the majority of plasma triglycerides. Chylomicrons are rapidly cleared from plasma as the preferred substrate of lipoprotein lipase. Accordingly, the postprandial increase in triglycerides is to a major extent accounted for by VLDL.

- In the fasting state, the increased triglyceride levels seen in conditions with high triglycerides are predominantly caused by VLDL production, rather than by limitations in clearance by lipoprotein lipase (with the exception of lipoprotein lipase deficiency seen in type I hyperlipidemia).

■ In hypertriglyceridemia, 70% of the increase in plasma VLDL triglyceride concentration is caused by an increased number of VLDL particles, and 30% is caused by triglyceride enrichment of VLDL particles. The majority of VLDL particles in hypertriglyceridemia leave the plasma before reaching the LDL density fraction, whereas most VLDL particles are converted to LDL particles in normolipidemic subjects. This is consistent with the normal to low LDL cholesterol levels seen in hypertriglyceridemia.

■ Triglycerides and Coronary Heart Disease

■ There has been considerable controversy as to whether elevated levels of plasma triglycerides constitute an independent risk factor for CHD.

■ As early as 1959, a case-controlled study showed an association between triglycerides and CHD. In a prospective study from 1965, an increased incidence of CHD among men with elevated triglyceride levels was demonstrated. However, even in these early studies, it was speculated that the association was not independent of other plasma lipids.

■ Several factors complicate the interpretations of studies investigating effects of triglycerides on CHD:
  ● Triglycerides have a wide day-to-day variation, and more than one measurement is preferable.
  ● The distribution of the triglyceride concentration in a patient sample is usually nonparametric.
  ● Triglyceride levels are strong determinants of HDL levels; that is, subjects with high triglycerides usually have low HDL cholesterol concentrations.
  ● High triglyceride levels are also associated with several other CHD risk factors, such as diabetes mellitus, insulin resistance, and obesity.

■ In a meta-analysis of population-based prospective studies (1998), based on 46,400 men and 10,800 women, each 1 mmol/L increase in fasting plasma triglyceride level was associated with a 32% increase in relative risk of cardiovascular disease in men and 76% increase in women. After adjustment for HDL cholesterol and other risk factors, the risks of cardiovascular disease decreased to 14% and 37%, respectively, but remained statistically significant.

■ A more recent meta-analysis, consisting of 10,158 cases among 262,525 participants, including the Reykjavik study and the EPIC-Norfolk study, concludes that there are moderate and highly significant associations between triglyceride values and CHD risk. However, with the associations depending on levels of other established risk factors, further studies are needed.

■ Recent large, long-term prospective studies from different populations confirm and support the role for triglycerides in CHD, particularly in the nonfasting (postprandial) state.

■ See Table 10-1.

Table 10-1:   Secondary Causes of Elevated Triglycerides

- Diabetes mellitus
- Obesity, overweight
- Physical inactivity
- High-carbohydrate diets
- Excess alcohol consumption
- Cigarette smoking
- Chronic renal failure
- Nephrotic syndrome
- Hypothyroidism
- Cushing syndrome
- HIV, lipodystrophy

■ Lipid-modifying Studies

- To establish that elevated triglycerides are of importance in the development of CHD, a beneficial effect of triglyceride-lowering treatment should be seen. However, there is a lack of primary or secondary prevention studies of individuals with isolated hypertriglyceridemia. The clinical benefit of reducing plasma triglyceride levels is predominantly studied in patients with either a combination of high triglycerides and low HDL cholesterol or, even more commonly, in patients with combined hyperlipidemia.

- The placebo-controlled primary prevention Helsinki Heart Study (HHS), enrolled middle-aged men with primary dyslipidemia (non-HDL-cholesterol ≥5.2 mmol/L). The largest lipid-lowering effect seen after gemfibrozil treatment was the 35% reduction of the triglyceride levels. After 5 years, there was a 34% reduction of nonfatal and fatal CHD in the gemfibrozil-treated group. The benefit was related to both a reduction of LDL cholesterol and an increase in HDL cholesterol, although the changes in these lipid levels were small. The most beneficial effect was seen in the group with elevated triglycerides and a high cholesterol:HDL ratio.

- In the placebo-controlled secondary prevention study Veteran Affairs High-Density Lipoprotein Cholesterol Intervention Trial (VA-HIT), men with low HDL cholesterol levels (<1.1 mmol/l) were included. After 1 year with gemfibrozil, triglyceride concentrations were 31% lower and HDL cholesterol 6% higher. Five years on gemfibrozil was associated with a 22% reduction in the risk of nonfatal and fatal CHD, as well as a significantly reduced risk of stroke.

- In the secondary preventive Bezafibrate Infarction Prevention (BIP) trial, patients with low HDL cholesterol (≤1.2 mmol/L) were treated with either bezafibrate or placebo. After a follow-up period of 6 years, the triglyceride levels were reduced by 21%. In contrast to gemfibrozil, bezafibrate treatment increased HDL cholesterol concentrations by 18%. Overall there were no significant effects of bezafibrate treatment, but a significant reduction in nonfatal and fatal CHD was observed in the subgroup of patients with baseline triglyceride levels ≥2.3 mmol/L.

- In the Bezafibrate Coronary Atherosclerosis Intervention Trial (BECAIT), men <45 years who survived a myocardial infarction were treated with bezafibrate or placebo for 5 years. There was less disease progression in focal lesions, and the cumulative coronary event rate was lower in the bezafibrate group, where triglycerides decreased by 31% and total cholesterol by 9%. HDL cholesterol increased by 9%, whereas LDL cholesterol did not change.

- Since 1994 several large clinical studies have demonstrated strong beneficial effects on CHD of treatment with 3-hydroxy-3-methylglutaryl coenzyme A (HMG CoA) reductase inhibitors (statins). Statins have become the cornerstone and primary choice for physicians in the treatment of hyperlipidemia, especially in patients with hypercholesterolemia and/or combined hyperlipidemia. However, in most of the statin trials, such as the primary preventive West of Scotland Coronary Prevention Study (WOSCOPS), the secondary preventive Scandinavian Simvastatin Survival Study (4S), the Cholesterol and Recurrent Events (CARE) trial, and Long-Term Intervention with Pravastatin in Ischemic Disease (LIPID) study, patients with high triglycerides either have been excluded or have failed to demonstrate any significant additive effects in subgroups of patients with high triglycerides.

■ Treatment of Elevated Triglycerides

- Secondary causes of hypertriglyceridemia should be ruled out.
- Alcohol restriction is recommended.
- Smoking cessation should be emphasized to reduce cardiovascular risk.
- Counseling with regard to dietary modification and performance of regular exercise represents the cornerstone of all approaches to lowering lipid levels.
- Consumption of a balanced diet favoring increased proportions of fruits, vegetables, fiber, seeds, and nuts, with reductions in total and saturated fat and cholesterol, should be encouraged. The caloric content of meals should also be addressed.
- Regular exercise should be encouraged for all. Daily exercise, in the form of brisk walking, swimming, jogging, or cycling, for a duration of 30 minutes, in order to build up a sweat and raise the heart rate, is recommended. This is a level of activity that most subjects should be able to achieve.
- Lifestyle modification, including physical exercise, will typically result in reductions in weight and waist circumference, with associated reductions in

LDL cholesterol and increases in HDL cholesterol, by up to 10%. More substantial reductions in triglyceride levels may be observed in overweight patients with hypertriglyceridemia at baseline.

- No clinical studies have been performed on preventing cardiovascular events in isolated hypertriglyceridemia.

- In combined hyperlipidemia, statin treatment is the cornerstone. Higher doses are often needed, especially to reduce triglyceride levels. Of the currently available statins, simvastatin, atorvastatin, and rosuvastatin are considered the most effective. The addition of fibrates, which is sometimes needed, may increase the ability to lower triglycerides. Combination treatment needs cautious monitoring and information on symptoms and increased risk of myopathies and rhabdomyolysis. This risk is increased when gemfibrozil is used and should therefore be avoided. Fenofibrate is the preferred fibrate choice in combination therapy in patients with high triglycerides and low LDL cholesterol.

- Fibrates reduce triglyceride levels through their action as peroxisome proliferators-activated receptor alpha (PPAR-α) agonists.

- Nicotinic acid (niacin) therapy, when used alone or in combination with statins for hypertriglyceridemia, increases HDL cholesterol and inhibits triglyceride production and reduces CHD risk. Niacin has also been shown to decrease LDL and VLDL levels. Niacin is recommended in combination with statins in patients with high triglycerides and low HDL cholesterol.

- Niacin therapy is associated with side effects that include flushing, palpitations, tachycardia, and nausea. Novel agents are on their way to reduce these side effects. A combination product with niacin and laropiprant, a novel flushing pathway inhibitor, was recently approved in the European Union, Norway, and Iceland and is undergoing clinical endpoint studies.

- Omega-3 fatty acids (fish oils) inhibit triglyceride synthesis involving PPAR agonism and direct effects on triglyceride production and VLDL secretion. Omega-3 fatty acids can be used as an adjunct to statins, niacin, and fibrates. Clinical trials with cardiovascular end points are needed.

- Patients with insulin resistance and/or metabolic syndrome (abdominal obesity, hyperlipidemia, hypertension, and impaired glucose tolerance/diabetes) often have combined hyperlipidemia. These patients are at high risk for cardiovascular disease/atherosclerosis and should be carefully taken care of. Their total cardiovascular risk and lifestyle interventions should be closely monitored, as well as pharmacological treatment against hyperlipidemia and hypertension.

- In extreme hypertriglyceridemia (>1000 mg/dL, 13 mmol/L), the major clinical risk is acute pancreatitis. These patients should be advised on a low-carbohydrate and low-fat diet, along with alcohol restriction, sometimes in combination with fibrate therapy.

- See Table 10-2.

Table 10-2:   Guidelines for Lipid Management According to Triglyceride Levels

Triglyceride level (mg/dL)	Primary lipid target	Therapeutic approach
<150	LDL cholesterol	Maintain healthy lifestyle.
150–199	LDL cholesterol	Physical activity and weight loss.
200–499	LDL cholesterol	Physical activity and weight loss, with consideration to initiation of drug therapy with a statin or addition of niacin/fibrate.
>499	Triglyceride	Implement very low-fat diet and alcohol cessation; optimize glucose levels, physical activity, and weight loss with consideration to use of niacin or a fibrate. Reducing risk of acute pancreatitis is critical in this scenario.

■ Summary

- There is increasing evidence that triglycerides contribute to the risk of developing CHD, particularly in the nonfasting (postprandial) state.
- The inverse relationship between triglycerides and other metabolic abnormalities complicates analyses of triglycerides' independent contribution to CHD.
- Lifestyle modification, including reduction in weight and waist circumference, is the cornerstone of treatment.
- Pharmacological treatment often includes combination therapy, with statins and other compounds, and needs to be monitored cautiously.

■ Suggested Reading

Assmann G, Schulte H, von Eckardstein A. Hypertriglyceridemia and elevated lipoprotein (a) are risk factors for major coronary events in middle-aged men. *Am J Cardiol.* 1996;77:1179–1184.

Austin MA. Plasma triglyceride as a risk factor for cardiovascular disease. *Can J Cardiol.* 1998;Suppl B:14B–17B.

Bansal S, Buring JE, Rifai N, Mora S, Sacks FM, Ridker PM. Fasting compared with nonfasting triglycerides and risk of cardiovascular events in women. *JAMA.* 2007;298:309–316.

Castelli WP. The triglyceride issue: A view from Framingham. *Am Heart J.* 1986;112:432–437.

Criqui MH, Heiss G, Cohn R, et al. Plasma triglyceride level and mortality from coronary heart disease. *N Engl J Med.* 1993;328:1220–1225.

Expert Panel on Detection, Evaluation, and Treatment of High Blood Cholesterol in Adults. Executive Summary of the Third Report of the National Cholesterol Education Program (NCEP) Expert Panel on Detection, Evaluation, and Treatment of High Blood Cholesterol in Adults (Adult Treatment Panel III). *JAMA.* 2001;285: 2486–2497.

Gotto AM, Jr. High-density lipoprotein cholesterol and triglycerides as therapeutic targets for preventing and treating coronary artery disease. *Am Heart J.* 2002;144:S33–S42.

Jeppesen J, Hein HO, Suadicani P, Gyntelberg F. Triglyceride concentration and ischemic heart disease: An eight-year follow-up in the Copenhagen Male Study. *Circulation.* 1998;97:1029–1036.

Lehto S, Rönnemaa T, Haffner SM, Pyörälä K, Kallio V, Laakso M. Dyslipidemia and hyperglycemia predict coronary heart disease events in middle-aged patients with NIDDM. *Diabetes.* 1997;46:1354–1359.

Mahley RW, Weisgraber KH, Farese RV, Jr. Disorders of lipid metabolism. In: Larsen PR, Kronenberg HM, Melmed S, et al., eds. *Williams Textbook of Endocrinology.* 10th ed. Philadelphia, Pa: Saunders; 2003:1642–1705.

Manninen V, Tenkanen L, Koskinen P, et al. Joint effects of serum triglyceride and LDL cholesterol and HDL cholesterol concentrations on coronary heart disease risk in the Helsinki Heart Study. *Circulation.* 1992;85:37–45.

Miller M. Differentiating the effects of raising low levels of high-density lipoprotein cholesterol versus lowering normal triglycerides: Further insights from the Veterans Affairs High-Density Lipoprotein Intervention Trial. *Am J Cardiol.* 2000;86(Suppl): 23L–27L.

Miller M, Seidler A, Moalemi A, Pearson TA. Normal triglyceride levels and coronary artery disease events: The Baltimore Coronary Observational Long-Term Study. *J Am Coll Cardiol.* 1998;31:1252–1257.

Nordestgaard BG, Benn M, Schnohr P, Tybærg-Hansen A. Nonfasting triglycerides and risk of myocardial infarction, ischemic heart disease, and death in men and women. *JAMA.* 2007;298:299–308.

Patsch JR, Miesenböck G, Hopferwieser T, et al. Relation of triglyceride metabolism and coronary artery disease. Studies in the postprandial state. *Arterioscler Thromb.* 1992;12:1336–1345.

Pejic RN, Lee DT. Hypertriglyceridemia. *J Am Board Fam Med.* 2006;19:310–316.

Sarwar N, Danesh J, Eiriksdottir G, et al. Triglycerides and the risk of coronary heart disease: 10,158 incident cases among 262,525 participants in 29 Western prospective studies. *Circulation.* 2007;115:450–458.

Szapary PO, Rader DJ. The triglyceride–high-density lipoprotein axis: An important target of therapy? *Am Heart J.* 2004;148:211–221.

Management of Specific Patient Populations

CHAPTER 11

Diabetes Mellitus

■ Background

- Diabetes mellitus is a metabolic disorder characterized by chronic hyperglycemia associated with impaired carbohydrate, fat, and protein metabolism, which is caused by defective insulin secretion, insulin resistance, and their combination.
- Type 2 diabetes mellitus accounts for 85% to 95% of all cases of diabetes, with an estimated prevalence in the general population of 2% to 6%.
- WHO (World Health Organization) has predicted that, in comparison with 1995, the global prevalence of type 2 diabetes will have more than doubled by 2025, affecting 300 million individuals. This global spread of diabetes mellitus is a major factor contributing to the prediction that cardiovascular disease will become the leading cause of death worldwide by 2025.
- In addition to the impaired glucose homeostasis seen in diabetes, concomitant hypertension and dyslipidemia influence the formation and progression of atherosclerosis.
- Coronary heart disease (CHD) is the most important cause of morbidity and mortality in patients with diabetes mellitus. The frequency of CHD is 3- to 4-fold higher in patients with diabetes mellitus type 2 than in those without it.
- More than two thirds of all the deaths in patients with type 2 diabetes mellitus are caused by macrovascular complications of the disease, such as CHD, cerebrovascular disease, and peripheral vascular disease.
- Patients with established atherosclerotic cardiovascular disease have a high risk of recurrent events. Accordingly, this patient cohort requires the most intensive risk factor modification. Increasing evidence has also highlighted patients with either type 2 diabetes mellitus or multiple risk factors (10-year Framingham risk >20%) as coronary risk equivalents. As a result, these groups also require intensive risk modification, even in the absence of established atherosclerotic disease.
- LDL cholesterol lowering, especially with statin therapy, is effective in reducing cardiovascular events in diabetes patients. However, a substantial residual risk of recurrent CHD remains, indicating that hypertriglyceridemia and low HDL cholesterol levels need to be addressed, requiring the development of new therapeutic options and strategies.

■ Diabetic Dyslipidemia

- In well-controlled type 1 diabetes, lipid and lipoprotein concentrations are similar to those in nondiabetic subjects.
- Poorly controlled type 1 diabetes is often associated with elevated levels of total cholesterol, triglycerides, VLDL, and chylomicrons and with decreased HDL cholesterol. The main determinants of dyslipidemia in type 1 diabetes are age, obesity, poor glycemic control, and nephropathy.
- The typical dyslipidemic pattern of type 2 diabetes is characterized by the presence of:
  - elevated triglycerides,
  - low HDL cholesterol, and
  - normal to slightly elevated LDL cholesterol, with an abundance of small, dense LDL particles.
- This typical diabetic phenotype is often referred to as the "atherogenic lipid triad."
- Triglyceride metabolism is impaired in patients with diabetes in both the fasting and the postprandial states, with chylomicrons, VLDL, and their cholesterol-rich remnants present in plasma longer and at higher concentrations than in nondiabetics.
- Elevated triglyceride levels are mainly caused by increased hepatic triglyceride synthesis, induced by an increased flux of free fatty acids (FFAs) to the liver. This increased triglyceride synthesis leads to increased VLDL production.
- There is also a delayed clearance of VLDL from plasma in patients with diabetes due to decreased lipoprotein lipase activity.
- Insulin normally inhibits the hepatic production of triglyceride-rich VLDL. This effect is attenuated in the insulin resistance state present in type 2 diabetes, contributing to hypertriglyceridemia.
- Plasma FFAs are increased in diabetes and obesity due to the reduced inhibitory effect of insulin on the fat-mobilizing lipolysis in adipose tissue. FFAs are continually mobilized from adipose tissue and are transported bound to albumin, with a high turnover.
- The proportion of small, dense LDL particles (type B LDL) is increased. These small LDL particles are considered more atherogenic than the large, buoyant (type A) particles. This corresponds to an increased number of apoB-containing lipoproteins, which, together with the increased VLDL levels, cause increased apoB concentrations, and this may contribute to the heightened cardiovascular risk seen in patients with diabetes, even though their LDL cholesterol is normal.
- In the presence of hyperglycemia, lipoproteins undergo qualitative modifications (such as glycation and oxidation), further increasing their atherogenic properties.

■ Management of Diabetic Dyslipidemia

Current Guidelines

- Diabetes mellitus is considered a CHD risk equivalent, putting the patients with diabetes in the high-risk group that needs aggressive lipid-lowering strategy.
- In the Third Report of the Expert Panel on Detection, Evaluation, and Treatment of High Blood Cholesterol in Adults (Adult Treatment Panel III), the primary target is to achieve LDL cholesterol <100 mg/dL (2.6 mmol/L), and there is an optional therapeutic goal of LDL cholesterol <70 mg/dL (1.8 mmol/L) for very high-risk patients, such as those with both CHD and diabetes.
- When triglycerides are >200 mg/dL (2.3 mmol/L), non-HDL cholesterol becomes an important target. Non-HDL cholesterol equals total cholesterol less HDL cholesterol, and the target for non-HDL cholesterol is 30 mg/dL (0.8 mmol/L) higher than for LDL cholesterol.
- If triglyceride levels are >500 mg/dL (6.6 mmol/L), there is a risk of acute pancreatitis, and patients should be medically treated.
- The American Diabetes Association (ADA) guidelines have similar LDL cholesterol goals to those of the National Cholesterol Education Program's (NCEP's) ATP III guidelines, but they also address a triglyceride goal of <150 mg/dL (1.7 mmol/L) and an optional HDL cholesterol goal of >40 mg/dL (1.15 mmol/L) in men and >50 mg/dL (1.3 mmol/L) in women. The ADA guidelines are similar to the joint European Association for the Study of Diabetes (EASD) and European Society of Cardiology (ESC) guidelines.
- In diabetes patients without known CHD, the goal is to reduce LDL cholesterol to 100 mg/dL (2.6 mmol/L) or to reduce LDL cholesterol by 30% to 40% with a statin; if patients are <40 years of age and have no other risk factor, they are considered to be at low risk.

Lifestyle Modification

- Initially, treatment for dyslipidemia is directed toward optimizing lifestyle. Of great importance is counseling on nutritional management with dietary modification and the performance of regular exercise.
- Dietary recommendations for patients with diabetes are similar to those given to the general population. Consumption of a balanced diet favoring greater proportions of fruits, vegetables, fiber, seeds, and nuts, along with a reduced intake of total and saturated fat and cholesterol, should be encouraged. The caloric content of meals should also be addressed.
- Smoking cessation should be emphasized to reduce cardiovascular risk.
- Regular exercise should be encouraged for all patients. Daily exercise is recommended, in the form of brisk walking, swimming, jogging, or cycling, for a duration of 30 minutes in order to build up a sweat and raise heart rate. Most people should be able to achieve this level of activity.

- These lifestyle modifications, if followed, will typically result in reductions in weight and waist circumference, with associated reductions in LDL cholesterol and triglycerides and increases in HDL cholesterol.

■ Medical Treatment

Statins

- Statins have been the most investigated class of therapeutic agents. Accordingly, substantial information has been collected with regard to their safety. Several landmark clinical trials of statins in primary and secondary prevention studies have demonstrated a 30% to 35% reduction in CHD event rate and a 25% to 45% reduction in LDL cholesterol levels. Substudies and post hoc analyses in diabetes patients have been performed in these large, randomized trials, but studies performed entirely in diabetic cohorts are scarce.
- The Heart Protection Study (HPS) evaluated simvastatin 40 mg in 20,536 high-risk patients with either established cardiovascular disease, diabetes, or treated hypertension across a broad range of LDL cholesterol levels. Included were 5963 patients with known diabetes, and after 5 years of follow-up, simvastatin was associated with a 22% reduction in the first major coronary event, stroke, or revascularization. A similar reduction of 27% was demonstrated in the 2426 diabetic patients who had LDL cholesterol <116 mg/dL (3 mmol/L) at baseline, implying that the benefit of statin treatment extends to much lower levels than previously observed.
- The Collaborative Atorvastatin Diabetes Study (CARDS) evaluated the impact of atorvastatin 10 mg in 2838 diabetic patients with an additional risk factor but with no known cardiovascular disease and an LDL cholesterol <160 mg/dL (4.14 mmol/L) and triglyceride levels <600 mg/dL (6.78 mmol/L). The study was stopped prematurely after 3.9 years due to a 37% reduction in cardiovascular events with atorvastatin. Assessed separately, acute CHD was reduced by 36%, coronary revascularizations by 31%, and the stroke rate by 48%. Atorvastatin also reduced the death rate by 27%, which, however, did not reach statistical significance ($p = 0.059$). Prior to this study, the role of lipid-lowering therapy with statins for the primary prevention of cardiovascular disease in diabetes was debated. However, these results demonstrated that statins are safe and well tolerated in this patient group and that statin treatment should be withheld only in subjects with a very low-risk profile.
- The Atorvastatin Study for Prevention of Coronary Heart Disease Endpoints in Non-Insulin-Dependent Diabetes Mellitus (ASPEN) evaluated the impact of atorvastatin 10 mg in 2410 diabetic patients either with LDL cholesterol <160 mg/dL (4.1 mmol/L) and no known coronary disease or with <140 mg/dL (3.6 mmol/L) and known coronary disease. No significant reduction in cardiovascular events was observed in any subgroup, although it was noted that

additional lipid-lowering therapy was initiated more often in placebo patients and the dropout rate in the study was high.

▫ The Scandinavian Simvastatin Survival Study (4S) assessed the impact of simvastatin 20–40 mg in 4444 patients with established coronary heart disease and total cholesterol 212–309 mg/dL (5.5–8.0 mmol/L). After 5.4 years of follow-up, a 35% reduction in LDL cholesterol was associated with a 30% reduction in total mortality, a 34% reduction in cardiovascular events, a 37% reduction in coronary revascularization, and a 28% reduction in stroke. The greatest impact was observed in patients with low levels of HDL cholesterol and hypertriglyceridemia at baseline. There were only 202 patients with known diabetes in this cohort, but analyses in this small subgroup showed that the absolute benefit of statin treatment was even greater than in the nondiabetic patients, due to the higher absolute risk of CHD in diabetes patients.

▫ Similarly, subgroup analyses from the major lipid-lowering trials with statins have demonstrated similar or even greater beneficial effects in reducing CHD risk in diabetes patients, in those both with and without prior cardiovascular disease. A meta-analysis of more than 90,000 patients enrolled in 14 trials of statin therapy revealed that each 40 mg/dL (1 mmol/L) reduction in LDL cholesterol was associated with an approximate 20% reduction in vascular events during 5 years of follow-up. In the 18,686 diabetic patients, a 21% reduction in events was observed.

▫ Statins, therefore, are considered the first-line lipid-lowering therapy in patients with diabetes. However, with the substantial remaining residual risk of CHD, addressing high triglycerides and low HDL cholesterol levels have potential impact. Additional therapy with fibrates or nicotinic acid to achieve lipid goals may be needed; the choice is often determined by tolerance and the side effect profile.

Fibric Acid Derivatives

▫ Fibric acid derivatives (fibrates) are peroxisome proliferator-activated receptor-α (PPAR-α) agonists. PPAR-α is a nuclear hormone receptor, which is involved in the regulation of HDL synthesis, reverse cholesterol transport, fatty acid metabolism, lipase activity, and inflammatory cascades.

▫ Fibrates are weak activators of the receptor, and the effects are seen as decreased triglyceride and non-HDL cholesterol levels, slightly decreased LDL cholesterol levels, and modestly increased HDL cholesterol. From a meta-analysis of randomized fibrate studies published before 2005, mean reductions of 36% in triglycerides, 11% in total cholesterol, and 8% in LDL cholesterol were reported, along with a 10% increase in HDL cholesterol levels.

▫ The Helsinki Heart Study (HHS) was a primary prevention placebo-controlled study with gemfibrozil in 4081 men with non-HDL cholesterol >200 mg/dL (5.2 mmol/L). After 5 years of follow-up, there was a reduction in CHD events of 34%. A subgroup analysis of the 135 patients with type 2 diabetes revealed a reduction of CHD events of 68%, but it was not considered statistically significant due to the small sample size.

- In the secondary prevention trial Veteran Affairs High-Density Lipoprotein Cholesterol Intervention Trial (VA-HIT), 2531 men with CHD and low HDL cholesterol <40 mg/dL (<1 mmol/L) were randomized to gemfibrozil or placebo. In the 627 subjects with diabetes, there was a reduction of 32% in cardiovascular events (nonfatal myocardial infarction, coronary deaths, and stroke), in comparison with an 18% event reduction in subjects without diabetes.

- In the secondary preventive Bezafibrate Infarction Prevention (BIP) study, 3090 patients with known CHD and specific lipid profile (triglycerides <300 mg/dL, LDL cholesterol <180 mg/dL, and HDL cholesterol <45 mg/dL) were randomized to bezafibrate or placebo and followed for 6 years. In spite of an 18% increase in HDL cholesterol and a 21% reduction in triglycerides, there was no overall significant effect in cardiovascular events. With the low event rate, there was no subgroup analysis of the 309 subjects with diabetes. However, in a post hoc analysis, obese subjects (BMI >30 kg/m^2) and subjects with triglycerides >200 mg/dL (2.2 mmol/L) were demonstrated to have a clear risk reduction in cardiovascular events.

- In the Diabetes Atherosclerosis Intervention Study (DAIS), 418 patients with type 2 diabetes were randomized to 200 mg fenofibrate/day or placebo and followed for 3 years. DAIS was an imaging atherosclerosis progression study, which demonstrated a significant 40% reduction in minimum lumen diameter and a 42% reduction in the percentage diameter stenosis in the bezafibrate group and a nonsignificant 25% reduction in mean segment diameter.

- In the Fenofibrate Intervention and Endpoint Lowering in Diabetes (FIELD) study, 9795 patients with type 2 diabetes were randomized to fenofibrate (200 mg/day) or placebo. After 5 years of follow-up, 2131 had clinical atherosclerosis. The primary endpoint (CHD death and nonfatal myocardial infarction) was reduced by 11% in the fenofibrate group, but the percentage did not reach statistical significance. There was, however, a significant reduction in nonfatal myocardial infarction (24%) and coronary revascularization (21%). The increased concomitant use of statins during the study complicates the evaluation of the actual fenofibrate effect. There was also an increase in homocysteine levels in the bezafibrate group, which is of unknown significance.

Nicotinic Acid

- Nicotinic acid inhibits lipolysis in adipocytes in a mechanism mediated by the recently identified nicotinic acid receptor (GPR109A). By reducing free fatty acid flux from adipose tissue to the liver, nicotinic acid reduces triglycerides and LDL cholesterol levels. HDL cholesterol can be increased by up to 35% with higher doses, which is likely to result from a combination of changes in production, remodeling, and metabolism of HDL particles. However, the exact mechanisms of niacin effects are not yet fully elucidated.

- Early evidence of clinical benefit was observed in the Coronary Drug Project, in which use of niacin reduced the incidence of nonfatal myocardial infarction and long-term mortality in patients with established coronary heart disease.
- In the HDL-Atherosclerosis Treatment Study (HATS), a niacin-simvastatin combination was associated with a significant 60% reduction of clinical events and a coronary atherosclerotic plaque regression. Only 16% of the 160 patients had diabetes and were not analyzed separately.
- In ARBITER (Arterial Biology for the Investigation of the Treatment Effects of Reducing Cholesterol) 2 and 3 studies, it was shown that niacin in addition to statin treatment retarded atherosclerosis progression in the carotid arteries in addition to causing a reduction of existing carotid intima thickness.
- Ongoing are two large studies with niacin in combination with a statin, and they include patients with diabetes. The AIM-HIGH trial includes patients with prior CHD and evaluates simvastatin alone versus simvastatin plus extended release niacin. In the HPS2-THRIVE study, the long-term effects of extended release niacin plus laropiprant, when added to statin therapy, will be evaluated.

■ Summary

- The prevalence of diabetes mellitus is rapidly increasing throughout the world, thereby significantly contributing to increased cardiovascular morbidity and mortality. The frequency of CHD is 3- to 4-fold higher in patients with diabetes mellitus type 2 than in those without it.
- Impaired glucose homeostasis, together with hypertension and dyslipidemia, influences the formation and progression of atherosclerosis in diabetes.
- The typical dyslipidemia associated with type 2 diabetes is characterized by elevated triglycerides, low HDL cholesterol, and normal to slightly elevated LDL cholesterol, with an abundance of small, dense LDL particles.
- Diabetes mellitus is considered a CHD risk equivalent, putting patients with diabetes in the high-risk group. The primary goal is to achieve LDL cholesterol <100 mg/dL (2.6 mmol/L), with an optional therapeutic goal of LDL cholesterol <70 mg/dL (1.8 mmol/L) for very high-risk patients.
- LDL cholesterol lowering with statins is effective in reducing cardiovascular events in diabetes patients. However, a substantial residual risk of recurrent CHD remains, indicating that elevated triglycerides and low HDL cholesterol levels need to be addressed. There is a need for the development of new therapeutic options and strategies.

■ Suggested Reading

Adiels M, Olofsson SO, Taskinen MR, Borén J. Diabetic dyslipidaemia. *Current Opin Lipidol*. 2006;17:238–246.

American Diabetes Association. Executive summary: Standards of medical care in diabetes—2009. *Diabetes Care*. 2009;32:Suppl 1:S6–S12.

Baigent C, Keech A, Kearney PM, et al. Cholesterol Treatment Trialist Collaborators. Efficacy and safety of cholesterol-lowering treatment: Prospective meta-analysis of data from 90,056 participants in 14 randomised trials of statins. *Lancet.* 2005;366:1267–1278.

Carlson LA. Nicotinic acid and other therapies for raising high-density lipoprotein. *Curr Opin Cardiol.* 2006;21:336–344.

Carmena R. Type 2 diabetes, dyslipidemia, and vascular risk: Rationale and evidence for correcting the lipid imbalance. *Am Heart J.* 2005;150:859–870.

Colhoun HM, Betteridge DJ, Durrington PN, et al. Primary prevention of cardiovascular disease with atorvastatin in type 2 diabetes in the Collaborative Atorvastatin Diabetes Study (CARDS): Multicentre randomised placebo-controlled trial. *Lancet.* 2004;364:685–696.

Collins R, Armitage J, Parish S, Sleigh P, Peto R. Heart Protection Study Collaborative Group. MRC/BHF Heart Protection Study of cholesterol-lowering with simvastatin in 5963 people with diabetes: A randomized placebo-controlled trial. *Lancet.* 2003;361:2005–2016.

Dayspring T, Pokrywka G. Fibrate therapy in patients with metabolic syndrome and diabetes mellitus. *Curr Athero Rep.* 2005;8:356–364.

Diabetes Atherosclerosis Intervention Study Investigators. Effect of fenofibrate on progression of coronary artery disease in type 2 diabetes: The Diabetes Atherosclerosis Intervention Study, a randomized study. *Lancet.* 2001;357:905–910.

Ginsberg HN. Efficacy and mechanisms of action of statins in the treatment of diabetic dyslipidemia. *J Clin Endocrinol Metab.* 2006;91:383–392.

Grundy SM, Cleeman JI, Merz CN, et al. National Heart, Lung and Blood Institute, American College of Cardiology Foundation; American Heart Association. Implications of recent trials for the National Cholesterol Education Program Adult Treatment Panel III guidelines. *Circulation.* 2004;110:227–239.

Guidelines on diabetes, pre-diabetes, and cardiovascular diseases: Executive summary: The Task Force on Diabetes and Cardiovascular Diseases of the European Society of Cardiology (ESC) and of the European Association for the Study of Diabetes (EASD). *Eur Heart J.* 2007;28:88–136.

Keech A, Simes RJ, Barter P, et al. FIELD study investigators. Effects on long-term fenofibrate therapy on cardiovascular events in 9795 people with type 2 diabetes mellitus (the FIELD study): Randomized controlled trial. *Lancet.* 2005;366:1849–1861.

Knopp RH, d'Emden M, Smilde JG, Pocock SJ. Efficacy and safety of atorvastatin in the prevention of cardiovascular end points in subjects with type 2 diabetes: The Atorvastatin Study for Prevention of Coronary Heart Disease Endpoints in non-insulin-dependent diabetes mellitus (ASPEN). *Diabetes Care.* 2006;29:1478–1485.

Krauss RM. Lipids and lipoproteins in patients with type 2 diabetes. *Diabetes Care.* 2004;27:1496–1504.

Stamler J, Vaccaro O, Neaton JD, Wentworth D. Diabetes, other risk-factors, and 12-yr cardiovascular mortality for men screened in the Multiple Risk Factor Intervention Trial. *Diabetes Care.* 1993;16:434–444.

CHAPTER 12

Chronic Kidney Disease

■ Background

- The incidence and prevalence of chronic kidney disease (CKD) is increasing, mainly as a result of an aging population and rapidly increasing incidence of diabetes mellitus. CKD affects 10% to 18% of the adult population in the Western world and is becoming recognized as a strong risk factor for cardiovascular disease and death.
- In recent years it has become evident that very early and otherwise asymptomatic stages of renal disease are also independent cardiovascular risk factors. Nearly 25% of the population has increased urinary albumin excretion rates, which have been demonstrated to predict an adverse cardiovascular outcome, even in the setting of normal blood pressure and glucose control.
- A high proportion of patients with CKD develop cardiovascular disease, and the magnitude of its consequent morbidity and mortality exceeds that of the need for dialysis.
- Creatinine levels are elevated in 26% of patients with ischemic heart disease and in 40% of patients with diabetes mellitus.
- There is limited data to guide the management of dyslipidemia in patients with CKD, largely due to the fact that very few patients with CKD have been included in large randomized prospective clinical trials with cardiovascular outcomes.
- Patients with CKD commonly have severe atherogenic lipid abnormalities, yet many of them are undertreated. Concerns regarding safety and the apparent lack of evidence of clinical benefit are often cited as reasons for undertreatment.
- Besides dyslipidemia, other components are involved in the premature development of atherosclerotic cardiovascular disease in CKD patients, such as:
  - hypertension,
  - anemia,
  - inflammation,
  - increased oxidative stress,
  - vascular calcification,
  - endothelial dysfunction,
  - decreased nitric oxide bioavailability,
  - abnormalities of mineral metabolism,

- sympathetic activation,
- renin-angiotensin-aldosterone system activation, and
- increased levels of oxidized LDL.

■ Lipid Abnormalities in CKD

■ Chronic kidney disease can cause secondary hyperlipidemia and aggravate a preexisting primary hyperlipidemia. From a lipid perspective, CKD can be divided into three groups according to lipid profiles:
  - Chronic kidney disease
  - Nephrotic syndrome
  - Lipid abnormalities after renal transplantation

Chronic Kidney Disease

■ Dyslipidemia is often evident in early stages of CKD and is caused by dysregulated lipoprotein metabolism. Changes in apolipoprotein levels are usually observed before actual changes in traditional plasma lipids.

■ The typical dyslipidemia in CKD is characterized by increased triglyceride levels (triglyceride-rich lipoproteins) and low HDL cholesterol, whereas LDL cholesterol levels are normal to slightly elevated.

■ Elevated triglyceride levels result from low lipoprotein lipase activity, which is due to a combination of decreased production and increased systemic levels of its endogenous inhibitor, apolipoprotein C-III.

■ The presence of low levels of apolipoprotein A-I and A-II, hypertriglyceridemia, and chronic inflammation results in low HDL cholesterol levels.

■ Although high levels of lipoprotein(a) are often observed in CKD, the contribution to increased cardiovascular risk is unknown.

Nephrotic Syndrome

■ Hypercholesterolemia is common in nephrotic syndrome, resulting from increased production and decreased catabolism of LDL cholesterol.

■ The large protein excretion in nephrotic syndrome stimulates synthesis of proteins by the liver, including apolipoprotein B, a large protein that is not excreted and that replaces albumin as an osmotic plasma component. Therefore, increased VLDL synthesis occurs initially in nephrotic syndrome, and, with remaining lipoprotein lipase activity, LDL is formed.

■ As nephrotic syndrome progresses, lipoprotein lipase deficiency appears, resulting in decreased hydrolysis of VLDL to LDL and elevated triglyceride levels. HDL cholesterol levels are normal or low in nephrotic syndrome.

Lipid Management in CKD

■ The National Kidney Foundation (NKF) has guidelines that recommend aggressive treatment of dyslipidemia in all CKD patients. The guidelines are based on the high risk of cardiovascular disease (CVD) in these patients and on the risk reductions achieved in the general population, together with the overall safety of pharmacologic treatment.

▪ The NKF and National Cholesterol Education Program Adult Treatment Panel (NCEP ATP) III provides similar guidelines that are applicable in stage 1 to stage 5 CKD, including renal transplant recipients. However, some differences exist.

▪ Given that CKD patients are considered to have a high risk of cardiovascular disease, a target LDL cholesterol level <100 mg/dL (2.6 mmol/L) and a non-HDL cholesterol <130 mg/dL (3.4 mmol/L) are recommended for all patients, including renal transplant recipients, regardless of glomerular filtration rate (GFR).

▪ In the NKF guidelines, there is no recommendation to further lower LDL cholesterol to <70 mg/dL (1.8 mmol/L) in patients with established cardiovascular disease, as suggested by the NCEP guidelines.

▪ Lifestyle modification with diet and exercise should be implemented in all patients as the first step in lipid management. Consumption of total and saturated fat, cholesterol, and trans fats should be reduced, the intake of fibers should be increased, and weight loss should be advised.

▪ When LDL cholesterol level is 100 to 129 mg/dL (2.6 to 3.4 mmol/L), pharmacologic treatment should be initiated after 3 months of lifestyle changes.

▪ See Table 12-1.

Table 12-1:   Dosing Modifications for Lipid-Lowering Drugs in CKD

Agent	GFR 60–90 mL/ min/1.73 m²	GFR 15–59 mL/ min/1.73 m²	GFR <15 mL/ min/1.73 m²	Notes
Atorvastatin	No	No	No	
Fluvastatin	No	Not defined	Not defined	↓ dose by 50% at GFR <30
Lovastatin	No	↓ to 50%	↓ to 50%	↓ dose by 50% at GFR <30
Pravastatin	No	No	No	Start at 10 mg/day for GFR <60
Rosuvastatin	No	5–10 mg	5–10 mg	Start at 5–10 mg/day maximum for GFR <30
Simvastatin	No	No	5 mg	Start at 5 mg if GFR <30
Nicotinic acid	No	No	↓ to 50%	34% kidney excretion
Cholestyramine	No	No	No	Not absorbed
Colesevelam	No	No	No	Not absorbed

Table 12-1:   Continued

Agent	GFR 60–90 mL/min/1.73 m^2	GFR 15–59 mL/min/1.73 m^2	GFR <15 mL/min/1.73 m^2	Notes
Ezetimibe	No	No	No	
Fenofibrate	↓ to 50%	↓ to 25%	Avoid	May ↑ serum creatinine
Gemfibrozil	No	No	No	NLA recommends 600 mg/day for GFR <60 and avoid use for GFR <15
Omega-3 FAs	No	No	No	

Key: ↓ = decrease; ↑ = increase; CKD = chronic kidney disease; FA = fatty acid; GFR = glomerular filtration rate; NLA = National Lipid Association.
Source: Adapted with information from the K/DOQI clinical practice guidelines.

Mild to Moderate CKD (Stage 1 to Stage 4)

- The evidence for management of lipids in patients with early stages of impaired renal function primarily comes from post hoc subgroup analyses of large secondary prevention clinical trials in patients with established atherosclerotic disease. Patients with GFR 15 to <30 mL/min/1.73 (stage 4) are almost exclusively excluded from these randomized clinical trials.

- The only prospective randomized trial in patients with mildly impaired renal function is the Prevention of Renal and Vascular End-Stage Disease Intervention Trial (PREVEND IT). In that study, 864 patients with microalbuminuria were randomized in a 2 × 2 factorial design to 20 mg fosinopril/placebo and to 40 mg pravastatin/placebo and followed for almost 4 years. The pravastatin arm resulted in a nonsignificant trend with a 13% reduction in cardiovascular death and hospitalization for cardiovascular causes. The event rate in the study was very low and the study therefore underpowered.

- The Cholesterol and Recurrent Events (CARE) study evaluated the impact of pravastatin 40 mg in patients with a previous myocardial infarction and plasma total cholesterol <240 mg/dL (average levels of LDL cholesterol 139 mg/dL at baseline). In 5 years of follow-up, a subgroup of patients (1700) with creatinine clearance <75 mL/min showed a 28% relative risk reduction and a 4% absolute risk reduction in the combination of coronary death or myocardial infarction. These results were similar to or even more pronounced than in the general study, where a significant relative risk reduction of 24% in the primary end point was achieved.

- In the Pravastatin Pooling Project, three placebo-controlled randomized trials with pravastatin (total 19,700 patients) evaluated the effects on the primary outcome times to myocardial infarction, coronary death, and cardiac intervention. The three studies were the West of Scotland Coronary Prevention Study (WOSCOPS), the CARE study, and the Long-Term Intervention with Pravastatin in Ischemic Disease (LIPID) study. Of the patients studied, 4491 had moderate CKD (GFR between 30 and 60 mL/min/1.73 m² body surface area). A similar result was obtained in the CKD patients as in those without CKD, where 40 mg of pravastatin was associated with a 23% reduction in the composite outcome over 5 years.

■ A subgroup analysis of 6517 patients with impaired renal function in the Anglo-Scandinavian Cardiac Outcomes Trial (ASCOT) showed that treatment with 10 mg of atorvastatin for 3 years resulted in a significant 39% reduction in myocardial infarction and cardiac death.

■ Fibric acid derivatives (fibrates) reduce plasma triglyceride concentration and modestly increase HDL concentrations. They are considered when triglyceride levels are >500 mg/dL (5.6 mmol/L) or in patients with mixed dyslipidemia, which is common in CKD. Safety concerns have been addressed in CKD since the drugs can cause a reversible increase in creatinine levels and are metabolized predominantly by the kidneys.

■ Gemfibrozil was associated with a 20% reduction in cardiovascular events in patients with GFR 30–75 mL/min/1.73 m² body surface area in the Veterans Affairs High-Density Lipoprotein Intervention Trial Investigators (VA-HIT) study.

■ The NKF recommends gemfibrozil as the fibrate of choice in patients with CKD. Combination therapy with a statin and a fibrate is possible, but it needs close monitoring due to increased risk of rhabdomyolysis in patients with CKD. A switch to fluvastatin could be considered.

■ The combination of statins with ezetimibe, omega-3 fatty acids, and niacin should also be considered.

■ See Table 12-2.

Table 12-2:   Summary of Statin Trials in the Primary Prevention Setting

Trial	Setting	Comparison	Effect on clinical events
4D	Diabetics on hemodialysis	Atorvastatin/placebo	No effect on cardiovascular events
PREVEND IT	Microalbuminuria with GFR ≥60	Pravastatin/placebo	No effect on cardiovascular events
Heart Protection Study	Subgroup analysis with elevated creatinine	Simvastatin/placebo	Decrease mortality or major vascular event
CARE	Subgroup analysis with GFR ≤75	Pravastatin/placebo	Decrease coronary heart disease death or nonfatal myocardial infarction

Table 12-2: Continued

Trial	Setting	Comparison	Effect on clinical events
ALERT	Renal transplant recipients	Fluvastatin/placebo	No effect on cardio-vascular events
AURORA	Hemodialysis	Rosuvastatin/placebo	No effect on cardio-vascular events
VA-HIT	Subgroup analysis with creatinine clearance ≤75	Gemfibrozil/placebo	Decrease in coronary death and nonfatal myocardial infarction
OPACH	Coronary disease on hemodialysis	n-3 polyunsaturated fatty acid/placebo	No effect on cardio-vascular events

Lipid Management in Stage 5 (GFR <15 mL/min/1.73 or Dialysis)

- A registry study of 3716 U.S. patients in dialysis (20% hemodialysis, 80% peritoneal dialysis) revealed low use of statins (10%), which were primarily given to those with coronary disease or diabetes. Despite the low use, statin use was associated with a 37% reduction in cardiovascular mortality.

- In Die Deutsche Diabetes Dialyse (4D) study, 1255 hemodialysis patients with type 2 diabetes mellitus were randomized to 20 mg of atorvastatin or placebo and followed for 4 years. Despite an LDL cholesterol decrease of 42%, there was only a nonsignificant relative risk reduction of 8% in the composite end point of cardiac death, myocardial infarction, and stroke. A lower rate of coronary intervention but a higher rate of stroke were observed in the atorvastatin group.

- Similar results were recently published from the AURORA trial (A Study to Evaluate the Use of Rosuvastatin in Subjects on Regular Hemodialysis: An Assessment of Survival and Cardiovascular Events). In 2776 hemodialysis patients assigned to 10 mg of rosuvastatin or placebo, no significant difference in the composite cardiovascular end point was demonstrated, despite a 43% lowering of LDL cholesterol with rosuvastatin.

- In the OPACH (Omega-3 Fatty Acids as Secondary Prevention Against Cardiovascular Events in Patients Who Undergo Chronic Hemodialysis) study, patients were randomized to 1.7g/day of omega-3 fatty acids or olive oil placebo. Although omega-3 supplementation did not lower the combined cardiovascular end point, a 70% reduction in myocardial infarction was observed.

- Further information on the effects of LDL cholesterol lowering in severe CKD will come with the results of the SHARP (Study of Heart and Renal Protection) study, where 3000 hemodialysis patients are randomized to 20 mg simvastatin alone/day or 20 mg simvastatin plus ezetimibe. This study will be presented in 2011.

- In patients in stage 5 CKD, atorvastatin and fluvastatin, with limited renal excretion, should be considered.

- In mixed dyslipidemia, the first line of added therapy should be omega-3 fatty acids.
- Recent guidelines discourage the use of fibrates, but, if they must be used, a reduced gemfibrozil dose of 600 mg/day can be given.
- Similarly, if niacin is used, a reduced dosing of <50% should be considered.

■ Renal Transplant Recipients

- Only one study has examined the benefits of a statin in renal transplant recipients. In the Assessment of Fluvastatin in Renal Transplantation (ALERT) study, 2101 patients were randomized to 40 mg fluvastatin or placebo and followed for 5 to 6 years. LDL cholesterol was decreased by 32%, but there was no significant effect on the combined primary end point of cardiac death, probable myocardial infarction, or coronary intervention.
- Special considerations need to be taken when patients are prescribed immunosuppressant therapies, which can lead to possible drug-drug interactions. Use of lower initial statin doses is currently recommended.

■ Summary

- Impaired renal function is increasingly common and associated with increased risk of cardiovascular morbidity and mortality.
- Lipid abnormalities are common in CKD, often with a mixed dyslipidemia pattern.
- Data from clinical trials is scarce, and the majority of studies are subgroup analyses from landmark clinical trials examining the effects of lipid lowering, in particular with statins.
- All patients should be treated aggressively to achieve at least LDL cholesterol levels <100 mg/dL (2.6 mmol/L) or lower, especially in patients with established atherosclerotic disease.
- Statins can be used safely in mild to moderate CKD (stages 1 to 3), but reduced dosing should be considered in later stages.
- Combination therapy needs close monitoring, but it can be handled. Reduced dosing is often needed.

■ Suggested Reading

Asselbergs FW, Diercks GF, Hillege HL, et al. Effects of fosinopril and pravastatin on cardiovascular events in subjects with microalbuminuria. *Circulation.* 2004:110:2809–2816.

Go AS, Chertow GM, Fan D, et al. Chronic kidney disease and the risk of death, cardiovascular events, and hospitalization. *N Engl J Med.* 2004;351:1296–1305.

Harper CR, Jacobson TA. Managing dyslipidemia in chronic kidney disease. *J Am Coll Cardiol.* 2008;51:2375–2384.

Heart Protection Study Collaborative Group. MRC/BHF Heart Protection Study of Cholesterol Lowering with Simvastatin in 20,536 High-Risk Individuals: A randomised placebo-controlled trial. *Lancet.* 2002;360:7–22.

Holdaas H, Fellstrom B, Jardine AG, et al. Effect of fluvastatin on cardiac outcomes in renal transplant recipients: A multicentre, randomised, placebo-controlled trial. *Lancet.* 2003;361:2024–2031.

K/DOQI clinical practice guidelines for managing dyslipidemia in chronic kidney disease. *Am J Kidney Dis.* 2003;41(Suppl 3):S1–S237.

Keech A, Simes RJ, Barter, P, et al. Effects of long-term fenofibrate therapy on cardiovascular events in 9795 people with type 2 diabetes mellitus (the FIELD study): Randomised controlled trial. *Lancet.* 2005;366:1849–1861.

Quaschning T, Krane V, Metzger T, Wanner C. Abnormalities in uremic lipoprotein metabolism and its impact on cardiovascular disease. *Am J Kidney Dis.* 2001;38:S14–S19.

Sarnak MJ, Levey AS, Schoolwerth AC, et al. Kidney disease as a risk factor for development of cardiovascular disease: A statement from the American Heart Association Councils on Kidney in Cardiovascular Disease, High Blood Pressure Research, Clinical Cardiology, and Epidemiology and Prevention. *Hypertension.* 2003;42:1050–1065.

Seliger SL, Weiss NS, Gillen DL, et al. HMG-CoA reductase inhibitors are associated with reduced mortality in ESRD patients. *Kidney Int.* 2002;61:297–304.

Svensson M, Schmidt EB, Jorgensen KA, Christensen JH. N-3 Fatty acids as secondary prevention against cardiovascular events in patients who undergo chronic hemodialysis: A randomized, placebo-controlled intervention trial. *Clin J Am Soc Nephrol.* 2006;1:780–786.

Tonelli M, Collins D, Robins S, Bloomfield H, Curhan GC. Veterans Affairs High-Density Lipoprotein Intervention Trial Investigators. Gemfibrozil for secondary prevention of cardiovascular events in mild to moderate chronic renal insufficiency. *Kidney Int.* 2004;66:1123–1130.

Tonelli M, Moye M, Sacks FM, Kiberd B, Curhan G. Cholesterol and Recurrent Events Trial I: Pravastatin for secondary prevention of cardiovascular events in persons with mild chronic renal insufficiency. *Ann Intern Med.* 2003;138:98–104.

Vaziri ND. Dyslipidemia of chronic renal failure: The nature, mechanisms, and potential consequences. *Am J Physiol Ren Physiol.* 2005;290:F262–F272.

Wanner C, Krane V, Marz W, et al. Atorvastatin in patients with type 2 diabetes mellitus undergoing hemodialysis. *N Engl J Med.* 2005;353:238–248.

Lipid Disorders in the Setting of HIV

■ Background

- Increased survival in response to use of antiretroviral therapy inevitably will result in a greater experience of chronic diseases such as atherosclerotic cardiovascular disease.
- Population studies have demonstrated a high prevalence of modifiable risk factors, including higher levels of triglycerides, lower levels of HDL-C, and higher rates of smoking in HIV-infected patients.
- A large number of studies of cohorts of HIV-infected patients demonstrated a variable relationship with cardiovascular risk, although many of the studies were small with relatively short periods of follow-up.
- The largest such studies demonstrated an increased risk of myocardial infarction in patients treated with protease inhibitors.
- A heightened cardiovascular risk in protease-inhibitor-treated patients who undergo interruption of therapy suggests that the lack of suppression of the viral load may also be important.
- As the length of average survival of HIV-infected patients increases, the relationship with cardiovascular risk will become increasingly apparent.

■ Assessment of Cardiovascular Risk in HIV-infected Patients

- Early development of risk factors warrants a high level of clinical surveillance.
- Initial assessment should determine the presence of hypertension, dyslipidemia, diabetes, family history of cardiovascular disease, smoking history, diet, and level of physical activity.
- Although conventional risk factor algorithms, such as Framingham, should be employed, these have not been validated in cohorts of HIV-infected patients.

■ Approach to Reduction of Cardiovascular Risk

- Lifestyle modification should be implemented in all patients as early as possible.
- Reduction in consumption of total and saturated fat and cholesterol, in addition to maintaining regular physical exercise, should be advised.
- Behavioral and pharmacologic approaches to smoking cessation should be actively pursued. Potential drug interactions between smoking cessation agents,

such as bupropion, and antiretroviral agents metabolized by cytochrome P450 should be considered.

- Pharmacologic intervention for management of dyslipidemia should be initiated in accordance with the National Cholesterol Education Program's (NCEP's) guidelines.
- Dyslipidemia requiring pharmacologic intervention will respond more favorably to initiation of lipid-modifying therapy than to replacement of a protease inhibitor with another agent such as a nonnucleoside reverse transcriptase inhibitor.
- Statins are typically the first-line therapy, unless triglyceride levels are greater than 500 mg/dL. Use of statins that are highly metabolized by cytochrome P450 3A4 (lovastatin, simvastatin) should not be coadministered with protease inhibitors. Although other statin agents can be used safely with protease inhibitors, the most experience has been with atorvastatin (partially metabolized by P450 3A4) and pravastatin. Because nonnucleoside reverse transcriptase inhibitors variably induce P450 3A4 metabolism, higher statin doses may be required, although doses should be titrated cautiously while monitoring for signs of statin toxicity.
- Fibrates are typically required when triglyceride levels are greater than 500 mg/dL and do not commonly have drug interactions with antiretroviral agents. Coadministration with statins may be required but must be done cautiously.
- Niacin may also be used as monotherapy or in combination with statins in the setting of mixed dyslipidemic states. Niacin was well tolerated in very small studies whose participants were pretreated with aspirin to reduce cutaneous flushing.
- Omega-3 polyunsaturated fatty acids (fish oils) can be used safely to lower triglyceride levels. Antiplatelet effects may be of value in the setting of potential hypercoagulability associated with HIV-seropositive status.
- Bile acid sequestrants may reduce absorption of antiretroviral agents and should therefore be avoided. In contrast, ezetimibe more selectively inhibits intestinal cholesterol absorption and is not associated with significant drug interactions.

■ HIV-associated Lipodystrophy

- Central fat accumulation and loss of peripheral fat are associated with the abnormalities of glucose and lipid metabolism typically encountered in patients treated with antiretroviral therapy. There are also patterns of predominant fat accumulation or atrophy or mixed features in different patients.
- Variable prevalence in different cohorts likely results from marked differences in terms of clinical characteristics and use of individual antiretroviral agents.
- Atrophy and accumulation of fat are likely to represent the manifestation of two distinct syndromes.

▪ Lipoatrophy involves loss of subcutaneous fat in a predominantly peripheral distribution (face, arms, legs, abdomen, buttocks), while preserving the remainder of tissue mass. There have been variable reports of association with increasing age, higher viral load, hepatitis C coinfection, and insulin resistance. The major risks for development of atrophy is use of reverse transcriptase inhibitors and duration of their use. Use of protease inhibitors as monotherapy is not associated with an increased risk of lipoatrophy.

▪ Fat accumulation in a central distribution (cervico-dorsal area, abdomen, breasts) is associated with excess visceral adipose tissue and is present in up to 40% of HIV-infected patients. It is also associated with increasing age, females, hypertriglyceridemia, greater baseline extent of fat, low-fiber diets, and longer use of antiretroviral therapies (both reverse transcriptase inhibitors and protease inhibitors).

▪ It is recommended that screening of the extent and distribution of fat be integrated into routine assessments of patients receiving antiretroviral therapies. Although computed tomography and magnetic resonance imaging of the abdomen can reliably distinguish subcutaneous and visceral adiposity, this is largely reserved for the research setting.

▪ Reported in association with use of both protease inhibitors and reverse transcriptase inhibitors is the full spectrum of deranged glucose metabolism, including impaired glucose tolerance, impaired fasting glucose, and frank diabetes, although the development of overt diabetes is uncommon in HIV-infected patients. It may result from direct interference with glucose uptake into cells or as a consequence of redistribution of adipose tissue, particularly in genetically predisposed individuals. Fasting plasma glucose should be evaluated at 1 and 6 months after commencement of new agents and screened annually in all HIV-infected patients. Subsequent management involves tapering antiretroviral dosing and standard antidiabetic therapeutic approaches where appropriate.

▪ The need for management of lipodystrophy will be determined by the degree of concern due to morphologic disturbance, discomfort, and associated metabolic derangement. Management of lipodystrophy will depend on the predominant pattern in each clinical setting.

▪ For lipoatrophy, consideration should be given to switching therapy from a thymidine analogue nucleoside to a nonnucleoside reverse transcriptase inhibitor. Thiazoladinediones have been used with some success, particularly in the insulin-resistant patient. Experimental use of pyrimidine nucleoside analogues and leptin are largely restricted to clinical trials at this stage. Fat replacement therapy by means of surgical techniques or reinjectable therapies can be used for cosmetic indications.

▪ Given that the association between HIV therapies and fat accumulation is less established, it is unknown whether switching agents is as beneficial as observed in lipoatrophy. Diet and exercise are critical in the management of fat accumulation. Metformin has been used in the setting of concomitant diabetes. Emerging data suggests that subcutaneous administration of human growth hormone or human growth hormone-releasing hormone may promote fat loss. Surgical techniques, such as liposuction and breast reduction, are also considered for cosmetic indications.

■ Summary

- With increasing longevity, a high prevalence of cardiovascular risk factors is found in HIV-infected patients.
- Abnormalities of lipid and glucose metabolism and fat accumulation are common.
- Many antiretroviral pharmacological agents contribute to these events.
- Patients should be screened for lipid and glucose abnormalities at baseline, at 6 months, and then annually after commencing therapy.
- Management includes altering drug doses and use of standard therapies for control of lipids and glucose.
- Drug interactions are important and should be considered.

■ Suggested Reading

Carr A, Samaras K, Chisholm DJ, Cooper DA. Pathogenesis of HIV-1-protease inhibitor-associated peripheral lipodystrophy, hyperlipidaemia, and insulin resistance. *Lancet.* 1998;351:1881–1883.

Dube MP, Stein JH, Aberg JA, et al. Guidelines for the evaluation and management of dyslipidemia in human immunodeficiency virus (HIV)-infected adults receiving antiretroviral therapy: Recommendations of the HIV Medical Association of the Infectious Disease Society of America and the Adult AIDS Clinical Trials Group. *Clin Infect Dis.* 2003;37:613–627.

Kaplan RC, Kingsley LA, Sharrett AR, et al. Ten-year predicted coronary heart disease risk in HIV-infected men and women. *Clin Infect Dis.* 2007;45:1074–1081.

Mallon PW, Cooper DA, Carr A. HIV-associated lipodystrophy. *HIV Med.* 2001;2:166–173.

Oh J, Hegele RA. HIV-associated dyslipidaemia: Pathogenesis and treatment. *Lancet Infect Dis.* 2007;7:787–796.

Riddler SA, Smit E, Cole SR, et al. Impact of HIV infection and HAART on serum lipids in men. *JAMA.* 2003;289:2978–2982.

Schambelan M, Benson CA, Carr A, et al. Management of metabolic complications associated with antiretroviral therapy for HIV-1 infection: Recommendations of an International AIDS Society-USA panel. *J Acquir Immune Defic Syndr.* 2002;31:257–275.

Stein JH, Hadigan CM, Brown TT, et al. Prevention strategies for cardiovascular disease in HIV-infected patients. *Circulation.* 2008;118:e54–e60.

Visnegarwala F, Maldonado M, Sajja P, et al. Lipid lowering effects of statins and fibrates in the management of HIV dyslipidemias associated with antiretroviral therapy in HIV clinical practice. *J Infect*. 2004;49:283–290.

Willig JH, Jackson DA, Westfall AO, et al. Clinical inertia in the management of low-density lipoprotein abnormalities in an HIV clinic. *Clin Infect Dis*. 2008;46: 1315–1318.

CHAPTER 14

Obesity and Metabolic Syndrome

■ Background

- Obesity and overweight are a increasingly prevalent healthcare challenge and have reached epidemic proportions in both developed and developing countries.
- It is estimated that worldwide more than 1.1 billion adults are overweight, of whom 312 million are obese.
- Abdominal obesity has rapidly increased, and in the United States 66% of the adult population is considered overweight and 34% are obese.
- Increased caloric intake, the shift from fiber-rich foods toward a Western diet with its increased consumption of refined carbohydrates, and physical inactivity have promoted this rapid increase in abdominal obesity, which is often accompanied by insulin resistance.
- In parallel with this global epidemic of obesity, the incidence of diabetes is estimated to rise by 72% in the United States and by 32% in Europe by 2030. However, the most dramatic increase in diabetes incidence (>150%) is predicted in the Middle East, Southeast Asia, India, Sub-Saharan Africa, and Latin America.
- The metabolic syndrome consists of a cluster of risk factors that are associated with insulin resistance and is a strong predictor of diabetes mellitus type 2.
- Abdominal obesity and the metabolic syndrome are associated with several metabolic disturbances and an increased prospective risk of atherosclerotic cardiovascular disease.

■ Clinical Definitions

- Overweight is defined as a body mass index (BMI) of 25.0 to 29.9 kg/m^2, and obesity is defined as BMI ≥30.0 kg/m^2. Extreme obesity is defined as BMI ≥40 kg/m^2.
- Other measures used to assess obesity include waist circumference and waist-to-hip ratio (WHR).

■ Several groups have characterized the metabolic syndrome, choosing risk factors that are easily measured (see Table 14-1). The definitions from the World Health Organization, National Cholesterol Education Program Adult Treatment Panel III (NCEP ATP III), and International Diabetes Federation (IDF) vary slightly, but all identify a population of insulin-resistant individuals that need risk factor modification.

■ Because no single pathophysiological defect is identified in the metabolic syndrome, the definitions are a combination of causes and consequences of insulin resistance. There has been a considerable debate as to whether this risk factor clustering represents a true syndrome, with any incremental significance beyond that of its components. However, it is important that the debate not diminish the potential clinical importance of individuals who have an increased cardiovascular risk.

■ The typical dyslipidemic pattern of the metabolic syndrome and abdominal obesity is similar to the dyslipidemia seen in type 2 diabetes mellitus and is characterized by elevated triglycerides and low HDL cholesterol. Non-HDL cholesterol is elevated, and LDL cholesterol is normal to slightly elevated, with the abundance of small, dense LDL particles.

Table 14-1: Current Definitions of the Metabolic Syndrome

WHO (1999)
Insulin resistance, identified as:
Type 2 diabetes mellitus
Impaired fasting glucose
Impaired glucose tolerance
Abnormal findings of hyperinsulinemic euglycemic clamp
Plus any two of the following:
Hypertension ≥140/90 mm Hg
Plasma triglycerides >150 mg/dL
HDL cholesterol:
Men <35 mg/dL
Women <39 mg/dL
BMI >30 and/or:
Waist:hip ratio
Men >0.9
Women >0.85
Microalbuminuria

NCEP ATP III (2001)
At least three of the following five criteria:
Waist circumference:
Men ≥102 cm (≥40 in)
Women ≥88 cm (≥35 in)
Triglycerides >150 mg/dL*
HDL cholesterol:*
Men <40 mg/dL
Women <50 mg/dL
Hypertension ≥130/85 mm Hg*
Fasting glucose ≥100 mg/dL

IDF (2005)
Abdominal obesity, identified as:
Waist circumference:
European men ≥94 cm (37 in)
European women ≥80 cm (32 in)
Ethnicity-specific values for other groups
Plus any *two* of the following:
Triglycerides >150 mg/dL*
HDL cholesterol:*
Men <40 mg/dL
Women <50 mg/dL
Hypertension ≥130/85 mm Hg*
Fasting glucose ≥100 mg/dL

*Or taking medication for this risk factor. Note: To convert to mmol/L: for triglycerides, multiply by 0.0113; for HDL cholesterol, multiply by 0.0259; for glucose, multiply by 0.0555.

■ The Role of Adipose Tissue

- The anatomic location of adipose tissue accumulation is fundamental to the metabolic risk profile predicting future cardiovascular disease and type 2 diabetes mellitus. In particular, increased abdominal adiposity is associated with the metabolic syndrome, elevated triglycerides, low HDL cholesterol, and increased inflammatory activity.
- There is an increased lipolytic activity in visceral (omental) adipose tissue in relation to abdominal subcutaneous adipose tissue, which may represent differences in receptor expression and in adipocytokine secretion.

Table 14-2:   Metabolic Risk Factors

Metabolic risk factor	Clinical finding
Atherogenic dyslipidemia	Elevated triglycerides, VLDL-cholesterol, non-HDL cholesterol
	Decreased HDL cholesterol
	Small, dense LDL particles
Glucose intolerance	Increased fasting glucose, HbA1c
	Impaired glucose tolerance
Hypertension	Elevated blood pressure
Proinflammatory state	Increased WBC, hs-CRP, IL-6
Prothrombotic state	Increased fibrinogen, von Willebrand factor, PAI-1

- From being previously regarded as only storage of excess energy in fat, adipose tissue evidently has important features, acting as an endocrine organ, secreting several different adipocytokines, and being a site of inflammation.
- Adipocytokines significantly contribute to regulation of biological processes such as energy metabolism, insulin sensitivity and inflammation, immune responses, and vascular homeostasis.
- The excess fat deposition in the liver appears to be the main predictor of insulin resistance and atherosclerosis in obese individuals.
- Lipid deposition in the liver results in the generation of nonalcoholic fatty liver disease (NAFLD), which is associated with insulin resistance.
- See Table 14-2.

■ Management of Dyslipidemia in Obesity and Metabolic Syndrome

Lifestyle Modification

- Counseling on lifestyle measures, including dietary modification and performance of regular exercise, is the cornerstone of management.
- Consumption of a balanced diet favoring greater proportions of fruits, vegetables, fiber, seeds, and nuts with reductions in total and saturated fat and in cholesterol should be encouraged. The caloric content of meals should also be addressed. Many people consume infrequent, large-calorie meals. The implementation of a diet that includes more frequent consumption (every 4 hours) of lower-calorie meals provides a more balanced dietary intake during a 24-hour cycle.
- Regular exercise should be encouraged for all. The intensity of exercise required is often overestimated by subjects who lack motivation. Daily exercise is recommended, in the form of brisk walking, swimming, jogging, or cycling, for a duration of 30 minutes, in order to build up a sweat and raise the heart rate. Most people should be able to achieve this level of activity.

- These lifestyle modifications, if followed, will typically result in reductions in weight and waist circumference, with associated reductions in LDL cholesterol and increases in HDL cholesterol by up to 10%. More substantial reductions in triglyceride levels will be observed in overweight patients, who are more likely to have hypertriglyceridemia.
- In patients with impaired glucose tolerance, several clinical trials have demonstrated that insulin sensitivity can be improved and type 2 diabetes mellitus can be prevented or delayed with intensive lifestyle modifications.
- Smoking cessation should be emphasized.

■ Medical Treatment

- Few strategies for the management of obesity have yielded long-term success. The only weight-reducing therapy with long-lasting effects on both weight and dyslipidemia is bariatric surgery.
- The LDL cholesterol goal depends on the total cardiovascular risk profile of the patient. However, with a normal to slightly elevated LDL cholesterol, non-HDL cholesterol is often increased, and a statin should be considered for first-line therapy in most patients.
- With persistent elevations of triglycerides (>200 mg/dL) or low HDL cholesterol, nicotinic acid or fibrates should be considered. Omega-3 polyunsaturated fatty acids have been demonstrated to have favorable effects on lipid profiles; however, there has been no clear beneficial effect in clinical end point trials.
- A promising approach in the management of obesity was the development of an inhibitor of the endocannabinoid receptor type 1 (CB1), which is present in both the central nervous system and the peripheral tissues. Inhibition of CB1 receptors with the drug rimonabant resulted in reduced food intake and decreased body weight. Clinical studies showed improved lipid profiles with increased HDL cholesterol and decreased triglycerides, C-reactive protein, and glycated hemoglobin. Despite these favorable metabolic effects, use of rimonabant was not demonstrated to slow progression of coronary atherosclerosis. This apparent lack of efficacy, in addition to reports of adverse psychiatric effects, led to cessation of further clinical trials with the compound.
- Often needed is a multifactorial risk factor modification strategy, with simultaneous approaches for treatment of hypertension, diabetes/impaired glucose tolerance, and dyslipidemia.

■ Summary

- Inactivity and sedentary lifestyle contribute to the rapidly increasing global epidemic of overweight and obesity. Overweight and obesity can lead to metabolic abnormalities, insulin resistance, type 2 diabetes mellitus, and increased cardiovascular risk.

- Lifestyle modification is the cornerstone for treating these patients. The development of manifest diabetes mellitus in patients with impaired glucose tolerance can be prevented by intensive lifestyle management.
- In moderate- to high-risk individuals, lipid-modifying treatment is often indicated, and statin treatment is considered first-line therapy in most patients. Combination therapy addressing persistent triglyceride and HDL abnormalities may be necessary.

■ Suggested Reading

Dayspring T, Pokrywka G. Fibrate therapy in patients with metabolic syndrome and diabetes mellitus. *Curr Athero Rep.* 2005;8:356–364.

Grundy SM, Cleeman JI, Merz CN, et al. Implications of recent trials for the National Cholesterol Education Program Adult Treatment Panel III guidelines. *Circulation.* 2004;110:227–239.

Guidelines on diabetes, pre-diabetes, and cardiovascular diseases: Executive summary: The Task Force on Diabetes and Cardiovascular Diseases of the European Society of Cardiology (ESC) and of the European Association for the Study of Diabetes (EASD). *Eur Heart J.* 2007;28:88–136.

Haslam DW, James WPT. Obesity. *Lancet.* 2007;366:1197–1209.

Hill NJ, Metcalfe D, McTernan PG. Obesity and diabetes: Lipids, "nowhere to run to." *Clin Sci.* 2009;116:113–123.

Kern PA, Di Gregorio GB, Lu T, Rassouli N, Ranganathan G. Adiponectin expression from human adipose tissue: Relation to obesity, insulin resistance, and tumor necrosis factor-alpha expression. *Diabetes.* 2003;52:1779–1785.

Knowler WC, Barett-Connor E, Fowler SE, et al., for the Diabetes Prevention Program Research Group. Reduction in the incidence of type 2 diabetes with lifestyle intervention or metformin. *N Engl J Med.* 2002;346:393–403.

Mathieu P, Poirier P, Pibarot P, Lemieux I, Despres JP. Visceral obesity: The link among inflammation, hypertension, and cardiovascular disease. *Hypertension.* 2009;53:577–584.

Tuomilehto J, Lindstrom J, Eriksson JG, et al., for the Finnish Diabetes Prevention Group. Prevention of type 2 diabetes mellitus by changes in lifestyle among subjects with impaired glucose tolerance. *N Engl J Med.* 2001;344:1343–1350.

World Health Organization. *Obesity: Preventing and managing the global epidemic.* WHO technical report series 894. Geneva, Switzerland: WHO; 2000.

CHAPTER 15

Heart Failure and Transplantation

■ Background

■ Systolic heart failure resulting from ischemic and nonischemic cardiomyopathies is associated with considerable morbidity and mortality.

■ Although the benefit of lipid-lowering therapies has been established in populations without heart failure, clinical trials have not typically enrolled large numbers of patients with either clinical features of heart failure or severely impaired left ventricular systolic function.

■ Given that atherosclerotic cardiovascular disease is a leading cause of heart failure in Western countries, it is possible that the established benefits of lipid-modifying therapy on atherosclerosis may translate to an improvement in heart failure outcomes.

■ Rationale for Testing Effect of Statins in Heart Failure

■ Statins have been reported to possess a number of pleiotropic functional properties, including antioxidant and anti-inflammatory activities, in addition to having a beneficial effect on endothelial function. These functional properties may have a favorable impact both on the incidence of acute coronary syndromes due to plaque rupture, a precipitant of heart failure and decompensation, and also directly on myocardial function in patients with established heart failure.

■ Observational studies suggest that statin use is associated with improved outcome in patients with heart failure. This is supported by findings of small, prospective studies in patients with both ischemic and nonischemic heart failure that demonstrate an improvement in both systolic function and clinical outcome with statin use.

■ Given that heart failure was typically excluded in large placebo-controlled statin trials and that the effect of therapy on ventricular function was not reported, it remains to be conclusively determined whether statin use is beneficial in this cohort.

■ A number of observations from clinical trials raises some doubt as to the potential efficacy of statins in the heart failure population. Rates of myocardial infarction are relatively low in heart failure, and some studies have suggested that low levels of total cholesterol are associated with an adverse outcome, although this has not been substantiated by other investigators.

■ A number of potential harmful effects of statins in the setting of heart failure have been proposed. Lipoproteins may interact with endotoxin, which enters the systemic circulation from an edematous intestinal wall. Endotoxin may subsequently have a direct adverse effect on myocardial function. Decreased generation of coenzyme Q10 and an increase in production of selenoproteins may have a direct role in promotion of both skeletal and cardiac myopathy.

■ Clinical Evidence in Heart Failure

■ A meta-analysis of 11 retrospective clinical studies of more than 100,000 patients revealed that use of statin therapy was associated with a 28% reduction in mortality, with no difference in patients with ischemic and nonischemic forms of disease.

■ Small studies reveal that statins typically have a favorable effect on a wide range of biomarkers in patients with heart failure, including left ventricular dimensions and ejection fraction, flow-mediated dilatation, functional class, and systemic levels of both brain natriuretic peptide and markers of inflammatory activity.

■ The Cholesterol and Recurrent Events (CARE) study analysis of the subgroup with a left ventricular ejection fraction between 25% and 40% at baseline demonstrated a significant reduction in clinical events with use of pravastatin, with no evidence of heterogeneity compared with the entire cohort.

■ The Controlled Rosuvastatin Multinational Trial in Heart Failure (CORONA) directly tested the impact of administration of statin therapy in patients with systolic heart failure. The 5011 patients, greater than 60 years of age and with clinical systolic heart failure due to ischemic causes, were treated with rosuvastatin 10 mg or placebo. Despite a 45% reduction in LDL cholesterol and 37% reduction in C-reactive protein (CRP), treatment with rosuvastatin was not associated with a reduction in the composite endpoint of cardiovascular death, nonfatal myocardial infarction, or stroke. A beneficial effect was observed on the rate of hospitalization for cardiovascular causes. Although this study did not demonstrate a benefit, it established that statins can be administered safely in a heart failure population. Therefore, though the study suggests that statins should not be initiated specifically because a patient has heart failure, the tolerability suggests that statins can continue to be safely administered to the patient who requires statin therapy and who develops heart failure.

■ The Gruppo Italiano per lo Studio della Sopravvivenza nell'Infarto Miocardico Heart Failure (GISSI-HF) study will also investigate the impact of statin therapy in 7000 patients with symptomatic systolic heart failure and with at least one hospital admission for heart failure in the preceding 12 months. In contrast to CORONA, patients with either ischemic or nonischemic causes of heart failure will be enrolled. Nested within a study of the effect of omega-3 polyunsaturated fatty acid supplementation, patients will be randomized to treatment with rosuvastatin 10 mg or placebo. It is of considerable interest to determine whether inclusion of younger patients and nonischemic cardiomyopathy will result in a different outcome.

■ Lipid Disorders in Transplantation Recipients

▪ Dyslipidemia is common in patients following solid organ transplantation, with prevalence rates between 60% and 85% of patients. This is characterized by elevations of both LDL cholesterol and triglycerides. Although many patients with ischemic forms of cardiomyopathy have concomitant dyslipidemia prior to transplantation, lipid abnormalities typically occur in those with normal lipid profiles within 2 to 3 months following transplantation. Posttransplant increases in lipid levels are typically observed within 2 to 3 weeks and tend to plateau by 3 months, provided that there is no further weight gain.

▪ A number of factors influence the development of lipid abnormalities in the posttransplant period, including use of immunosuppressant therapy (steroids, cyclosporine, tacrolimus, rapamycin), diabetes, renal insufficiency, nephrotic syndrome, hypothyroidism, and male gender.

▪ Given the deleterious effect of steroids on glycemic and lipid control, minimally required doses should be used. The effect of cyclosporine and tacrolimus on LDL cholesterol levels appears to be dose dependent and, although the precise mechanism underlying the dyslipidemia remains to be defined, it has become apparent that, given its lipophilicity, cyclosporine circulates in the systemic circulation within LDL and HDL particles and may modify lipid metabolism. The adverse impact on lipid levels is more pronounced with cyclosporine than with tacrolimus. Rapamycin inhibits lipoprotein lipase activity, resulting in reduced renal excretion of apoB-containing lipoproteins and hypertriglyceridemia.

■ Management of Lipids in Transplant Recipients

▪ Given the prevalence of underlying atherosclerotic disease and risk of incident allograft vasculopathy, intensive lipid modification is warranted in all solid organ transplant recipients.

▪ Lifestyle measures with diet and exercise remain the cornerstone of approaches to control of lipids. Referral to a rehabilitation program is typically routine in the postoperative management of heart transplant recipients.

▪ The pharmacologic approach to management of lipid disorders is similar to that used in the nontransplant patient, with the important caveat that high vigilance is required for potential drug interactions with immunosuppressive therapy.

▪ Many statins and fibrates are metabolized by cytochrome P450 3A4, a metabolic pathway inhibited by cyclosporine and tacrolimus, and should therefore be used with caution given the risk of myopathy. Consideration should be given to the use of statins that are not metabolized by this pathway, such as pravastatin. Elevations in liver enzymes are more typically encountered with niacin when coadministered with cyclosporine and azathioprine. Because bile acid sequestrants can modify intestinal absorption of fat-soluble medications, such as cyclosporine, drug levels should be monitored closely. Furthermore, ezetimibe is not typically used in transplant recipients due to observations that interactions with cyclosporine raise ezetimibe levels by 2- to 12-fold. Fish oils are well tolerated and should be considered in the setting of hypertriglyceridemia.

- Attention should also focus on the ideal immunosuppressant therapy. Using minimal steroid doses and substituting tacrolimus for cyclosporine can have favorable effects on LDL cholesterol and triglyceride levels. At all times the impact of changing therapies to reduce the risk of atherosclerotic disease, transplant vasculopathy, or pancreatitis should be balanced against the need to prevent organ rejection.

■ Lipid Treatment and Prevention of Transplant Vasculopathy

- Development of vasculopathy is a leading cause of the need for repeat transplantation, morbidity, and mortality in organ transplant recipients following the first year.
- The high incidence of hypercholesterolemia in cardiac transplant recipients results in the likelihood that the majority of patients will require lipid-lowering therapy.
- Several small, prospective clinical trials have demonstrated that administration of statin therapy in heart transplant recipients is accompanied by a reduced incidence and progression of transplant vasculopathy and the associated survival benefit. As a result, statin administration is recommended for all heart transplant recipients, unless otherwise contraindicated.
- The anti-inflammatory, immunomodulatory, and endothelial effects of statins are likely to contribute to, besides lipid lowering, a beneficial impact on vasculopathy.

■ Summary

- Use of statins to specifically treat heart failure has not been associated with clinical benefit.
- Use of statins for management of ischemic risk in patients with heart failure is safe.
- Management of dyslipidemia in transplantation is essential.

■ Suggested Reading

Davidson M. Considerations in the treatment of dyslipidemia associated with chronic kidney failure and renal transplantation. *Prev Cardiol*. 2005;8:244–249.

Deedwania PC, Javed U. Statins in heart failure. *Cardiol Clin*. 2008;26:573–587.

GISSI Heart Failure Investigators, Tavazzi L, Maggioni AP, et al. Effect of rosuvastatin in patients with chronic heart failure (the GISSI-HF trial): A randomised, double-blind, placebo-controlled trial. *Lancet*. 2008;372:1231–1239.

Kjekshus J, Apetrei E, Barrios V, et al. Rosuvastatin in older patients with systolic heart failure. *N Engl J Med*. 2007;357:2248–2261.

Kobashigawa JA. Statins and cardiac allograft vasculopathy after heart transplantation. *Semin Vasc Med*. 2004;4:401–406.

Krum H, McMurray JJ. Statins and chronic heart failure: Do we need a large-scale outcome trial? *J Am Coll Cardiol*. 2002;39:1567–1573.

Massy ZA. Hyperlipidemia and cardiovascular disease after organ transplantation. *Transplantation*. 2001;72:S13–S15.

Wenke K. Management of hyperlipidaemia associated with heart transplantation. *Drugs*. 2004;64:1053–1068.

Role of Imaging Modalities

CHAPTER 16

Imaging

■ Background

■ Technological advances in arterial wall imaging permit visualization of the full extent of atherosclerosis in multiple vascular territories.

■ Serial in vivo imaging enables evaluation of the impact of clinical characteristics on the natural history of disease progression.

■ Arterial imaging has been employed to assess the influence of medical therapies that modify lipid levels.

■ Imaging Modalities

■ Coronary angiography has been used since 1958 to detect and quantify the extent of obstructive coronary artery disease. Angiography guides the use of medical and revascularization strategies. The number of diseased vessels predicts the subsequent incidence of clinical events in large registries. The presence of multivessel disease indicates patients who are likely to benefit from bypass surgery. However, angiography is limited as it:
  * requires an invasive procedure,
  * yields images of the lumen, not the vessel wall, and
  * provides no information on plaque composition.

■ Noninvasive ultrasonic imaging permits measurement of intimal-medial thickness (IMT) in the carotid and femoral arteries. Increasing carotid IMT is associated with risk factors, atherosclerosis in other vascular territories, and clinical events. This type of imaging:
  * can be applied in large populations spanning a broad range of cardiovascular risk,
  * detects early changes in the artery wall, although it is unclear if this advances to mature atherosclerosis at the specific site, but
  * provides no volumetric or composition information.

■ Intravascular ultrasound (IVUS) places a high-frequency ultrasound transducer in close proximity to the endothelial surface, generating high-resolution images of the entire vessel wall. Imaging throughout the length of an arterial segment
  * permits precise volumetric measurement of the extent of disease,

- characterizes the remodeling pattern of the artery wall and the multifocal nature of plaque rupture in the setting of acute coronary syndromes, requires an invasive procedure, and
  - provides a limited characterisation of plaque composition.
- Early data suggests that disease progression is greater in patients who experience a clinical event.
- Increasing resolution permits visualization of the coronary arteries by computer tomography (CT). Detection and quantitation of coronary calcification by CT correlate with the extent of coronary artery disease and prospective risk of clinical events. CT detects lumen stenoses, with particular accuracy in saphenous vein grafts. Limitations include radiation exposure, requirement for heart rate control, and intravenous contrast. Imaging is poor in regions containing stents. Ongoing technological advances, which improve imaging resolution, may permit visualization of plaque within the vessel wall.
- Magnetic resonance (MR) characterizes the extent and composition of atherosclerosis in the aorta and carotid arteries. Suboptimal resolution currently limits precise imaging in the coronary arteries. Advances in intravascular imaging, supported by the use of vascular coils, may permit coronary imaging.
- A number of novel intravascular modalities provide alternative techniques for characterization of coronary atherosclerosis. Optical coherence tomography (OCT) detects reflected light and generates a high-resolution image of the artery wall. OCT detects the degree of inflammatory activity within plaque and measures the thickness of the fibrous cap. OCT is limited by the need for invasive procedure, limited tissue penetration, and the requirement for saline flushing due to inability of imaging in blood. Palpography and elastography determine strain of fibrous caps overlying atherosclerotic plaque. Thermography is reported to demonstrate increased temperature at the site of inflamed, vulnerable plaques. Development of molecular-targeted imaging enables the characterization of pathological cascades involved in plaque formation and rupture.
- Arterial wall imaging modalities are summarized in Table 16-1 (page 136).

■ Impact of Lipid-modifying Therapies: Lessons from Arterial Wall Imaging

Lowering LDL Cholesterol

- Direct relationships have been observed between levels of LDL cholesterol and rate of disease progression in serial studies using angiography, carotid IMT, and IVUS.
- Early studies revealed that lowering LDL cholesterol either with cholestyramine in the National Heart, Lung and Blood Institute Type II Coronary Intervention Study and St Thomas' Atherosclerosis Regression Study (STARS) or with partial ileal bypass surgery in the Program on the Surgical Control of the Hyperlipidemias (POSCH) slowed progression of angiographic disease.

- Despite anecdotal reports of angiographic regression, randomized controlled trials failed to demonstrate an incremental benefit of LDL apheresis, in addition to background medical therapy.
- A large number of studies of statin therapy revealed a direct relationship between achieved levels of LDL cholesterol and the rate of progression of obstructive disease. The effect of statin therapy on disease progression appeared to be minimal compared with their impact on clinical events. No study demonstrated angiographic regression with use of statin monotherapy.
- A similar direct relationship is observed between the degree of lowering of LDL cholesterol and slowing the progression of carotid IMT. Carotid ultrasound demonstrated an incremental benefit of intensive versus moderate lipid lowering on progression of IMT. IMT regression was observed with intensive lowering of LDL cholesterol in cohorts with familial hypercholesterolemia in the Atorvastatin Versus Simvastatin Atherosclerosis Progression (ASAP) study and with dyslipidemia, meeting the criteria for lipid-lowering therapy in the Arterial Biology for the Investigation of the Treatment Effects of Reducing Cholesterol (ARBITER) study.
- The benefits of high-dose statin therapy have recently been extended to subjects who do not typically meet criteria for lipid-modifying therapy. In the Measuring Effects on Intima-Media Thickness: an Evaluation of Rosuvastatin (METEOR) study, low-risk subjects with modest hypercholesterolemia and evidence of intimal-medial thickening demonstrated halting of IMT progression in association with lowering LDL cholesterol to 78 mg/dL in response to rosuvastatin 20 mg daily. This finding also suggests that vascular imaging may identify patients likely to benefit from risk factor modification.
- The lack of effect of incremental lowering of LDL cholesterol on carotid IMT progression in the Ezetimibe and Simvastatin in Hypercholesterolemia Enhances Atherosclerosis Regression (ENHANCE) study has prompted speculation that different therapeutic strategies for lowering LDL cholesterol may have variable effects on the disease process in the artery wall. The reason for the lack of efficacy remains uncertain. The finding that baseline IMT was within normal limits and that the rate of progression was substantially less than previously observed in familial hypercholesterolemia suggests that use of lipid-modifying treatment in these patients may have altered the natural history of disease progression. The effect of this therapeutic approach on progression of coronary atherosclerosis and its impact on clinical events remain to be determined. Given the lack of proven efficacy, it is likely that use of ezetimibe will be reserved for patients who have not achieved their LDL cholesterol goal, despite use of maximally tolerated doses of other agents.
- An incremental benefit of intensive versus moderate lowering of LDL cholesterol was also observed on progression of coronary atherosclerosis, monitored by serial IVUS. In the Reversal of Atherosclerosis with Aggressive Lipid Lowering (REVERSAL) study, intensive lowering of LDL cholesterol to 79 mg/dL with

atorvastatin 80 mg daily halted progression of atheroma volume. Direct relationships between changes in atheroma volume and either LDL cholesterol or CRP
suggested that the benefit of high-dose statin therapy on disease is likely to
result from both lipid and nonlipid properties. More recently, A Study to Evaluate the Effect of Rosuvastatin on Intravascular Ultrasound-Derived Coronary
Atheroma Burden (ASTEROID) revealed that lowering LDL cholesterol to
60.8 mg/dL and raising HDL cholesterol by 14.7% with rosuvastatin 40 mg daily
promoted atheroma regression. Angiographic regression was also observed.
A pooled analysis of four clinical trials revealed that both LDL cholesterol lowering and HDL cholesterol raising independently predicted the benefit of statin
therapy on plaque progression. Accordingly, the change in apoB:A-I ratio, reflecting the balance of atherogenic and protective lipid particles, is the strongest
predictor of the benefit of statin therapy.

- Case reports and clinical trials have also demonstrated evidence of disease
regression on IVUS in response to treatment with LDL apheresis.
- More recent studies reveal that statin therapy reduces the lipid component and
raises the fibrotic component of coronary atherosclerosis, evaluated by radio
frequency analysis of IVUS. This is consistent with histopathology studies
demonstrating that statin administration is associated with a more stable plaque
phenotype.
- Despite early evidence that cerivastatin slows progression of coronary calcification, two subsequent randomized controlled trials failed to demonstrate a benefit of intensive versus moderate lipid lowering. These findings contrast with
the unequivocal benefit of this therapeutic approach on atheroma volume in
IVUS trials and highlights a potential discord between evaluating the potential
efficacy of agents with regard to their ability to slow progression of calcification. Furthermore, it challenges the concept that an increased burden of calcification may be a suitable approach to identify patients who are more likely to
derive benefit from use of medical therapies.
- Magnetic resonance imaging has demonstrated atheroma regression in the
carotid artery and aorta. In the Outcome of Rosuvastatin Treatment on Carotid
Artery Atheroma: a Magnetic Resonance Imaging Observation (ORION) study,
lowering LDL cholesterol with rosuvastatin had a beneficial impact on disease
progression and the size of the lipid-rich necrotic core.

Fibrate Therapy

- In the Bezafibrate Coronary Atherosclerosis Intervention Trial (BECAIT),
administration of bezafibrate to middle-aged males with a history of myocardial
infarction and dyslipidemia attenuated the reduction in minimum lumen
diameter on angiography.
- The benefits of fibrates were extended to diabetic patients in the Diabetes
Atherosclerosis Intervention Study (DAIS), in whom micronized fenofibrate
slowed angiographic disease progression.

- A similar benefit in slowing carotid IMT progression in diabetics was observed with administration of the PPAR-γ agonist, pioglitazone, in the Carotid Intima-Media Thickness in Atherosclerosis Using Pioglitazone (CHICAGO) study. Although pioglitazone-treated patients demonstrated more optimal glycemic control than those treated with glimepiride, the 15% increase in HDL cholesterol levels was demonstrated to be the strongest predictor of the benefit of pioglitazone on disease progression.
- More recently, the Pioglitazone Effect on Regression of Intravascular Sonographic Coronary Obstruction Prospective Evaluation (PERISCOPE) study confirmed these observations by demonstrating that a 16% increase in HDL cholesterol, a 15% reduction in triglyceride, and a 45% decrease in CRP were associated with halting progression of coronary atherosclerosis, evaluated by IVUS.

Niacin Therapy

- The combination of lowering LDL cholesterol and raising HDL cholesterol resulted in disease regression on coronary angiography in the HDL-Atherosclerosis Treatment Study (HATS). Disease regression was associated with a significant reduction in clinical events. This is the only robust evidence of disease regression on angiography with medical therapy. This benefit is lost in the presence of concomitant use of antioxidant vitamins.
- A similar benefit of niacin was observed with slowing carotid IMT progression in the Arterial Biology for the Investigation of the Treatment Effects of Reducing Cholesterol (ARBITER) 2 study. Raising HDL cholesterol, by the addition of extended-release niacin to simvastatin in males with established coronary artery disease, halted IMT progression. With ongoing therapy, regression of IMT was observed.
- The impact of niacin formulations designed to reduce the intolerance due to flushing has yet to be evaluated by arterial wall imaging.

HDL Infusional Therapy

- IVUS has characterized a rapid and beneficial impact of infusing reconstituted HDL on coronary atherosclerosis in humans. This supports early data demonstrating that similar infusions improved endothelial function and enhanced fecal sterol excretion, a surrogate marker of reverse cholesterol transport.
- In a study of 57 patients within 2 weeks of an acute coronary syndrome, weekly infusions of reconstituted-HDL-containing recombinant human apolipoprotein apoA-I Milano for 5 weeks promoted rapid coronary atheroma regression. The most profound regression was observed in the 10-mm segments that contained the greatest amount of plaque at baseline, suggesting that rapid mobilization of lipid could be achieved from lipid-rich pools within the artery wall.
- In a similar study design, infusing reconstituted HDL containing wild-type human apolipoprotein AI weekly for 4 weeks promoted a strong trend toward plaque

regression. An associated increase in plaque echogenicity suggested that infusional therapy could favorably modify plaque composition.

■ The potential benefit of infusing lipid-poor forms of HDL has stimulated interest in the development of techniques that permit selective delipidation of a patient's own HDL, which is then subsequently reinfused. A preliminary report from a small pilot study demonstrated evidence of atheroma regression in patients who received intravenous infusions of delipidated HDL.

■ The impact of infusional therapy on clinical outcome has yet to be evaluated in randomized clinical trials.

Cholesteryl Ester Transfer Protein (CETP) Inhibition

■ Substantial elevation of HDL cholesterol, in addition to incremental lowering of LDL cholesterol, in statin-treated patients with the CETP inhibitor torcetrapib did not slow carotid IMT progression in the Rating Atherosclerotic Disease Changes by Imaging with a New Cholesteryl-Ester-Transfer Protein Inhibitor (RADIANCE) 1 and 2 studies, conducted in the setting of familial hypercholesterolemia and mixed dyslipidemia, respectively.

■ A similar lack of efficacy of torcetrapib on progression of coronary atherosclerosis was observed using intravascular ultrasound in the Investigation of Lipid Level Management Using Coronary Ultrasound to Assess Reduction of Atherosclerosis by CETP Inhibition and HDL Elevation (ILLUSTRATE). The lack of slowing plaque progression was discordant with what would be predicted on the basis of both the substantial elevation of HDL cholesterol by 61% and achieved level of LDL cholesterol of 71 mg/dL. Subsequent analysis revealed an indirect relationship between achieved levels of HDL cholesterol and plaque progression, with regression observed in patients achieving high levels of HDL cholesterol with torcetrapib. This finding suggested that the HDL particles generated with CETP inhibition in humans are functional. The loss of this benefit in patients with low systemic potassium levels is consistent with recent observations that torcetrapib activates the renin-angiotensin-aldosterone axis. This off-target toxicity may have mitigated any potential benefit of raising HDL cholesterol and suggests that another CETP inhibitor, without such adverse effects, may be clinically efficacious.

Acyl:cholesterol Acyltransferase (ACAT) Inhibition

■ Uptake of esterified cholesterol by macrophages to become foam cells is one of the pivotal stages in plaque formation and propagation. Inhibition of acyl-coenzyme A:cholesterol acyltransferase (ACAT) has a profound beneficial impact on lesions in animal models of atherosclerosis.

■ Administration of the ACAT inhibitor, avasimibe, did not slow coronary plaque progression in the Avasimibe and Progression of coronary Lesions assessed by intravascular Ultrasound (A-PLUS) study. It was postulated that the lack of efficacy was due to the observation that avasimibe induced statin metabolism, resulting in higher levels of LDL cholesterol.

- In a subsequent study of an ACAT inhibitor without an effect on statin metabolism, a lack of benefit on plaque progression was also observed. In the ACAT Intravascular Atherosclerosis Treatment Evaluation (ACTIVATE), greater progression was observed in patients treated with the ACAT inhibitor, pactimibe. A potential proatherogenic influence of ACAT inhibition may result from cytotoxicity in response to increases in intracellular levels of free cholesterol.

Endocannabinoid Receptor Antagonists

- These therapeutic agents were developed to promote weight loss in the setting of abdominal obesity. Early clinical studies demonstrate that loss of abdominal adiposity is associated with favorable effects on levels of metabolic factors (triglyceride, HDL cholesterol, insulin resistance), blood pressure, inflammatory markers, and adipocytokines.
- The Strategy to Reduce Atherosclerosis Development Involving Administration of Rimonabant—the Intravascular Ultrasound Study (STRADIVARIUS) compared the effects of rimonabant and placebo, in addition to established medical therapy, in patients with abdominal obesity and coronary artery disease. Despite a 22% increase in HDL cholesterol, a 20% reduction in triglycerides, a 50% reduction in CRP, and improvement in glycemic control, the use of rimonabant did not significantly slow progression of the primary end point. The findings of a benefit with regard to the secondary end point, the change in total atheroma volume, and in the subgroup with hypertriglyceridemia at baseline suggest that this therapeutic approach may be of utility in abdominally obese patients who have associated metabolic abnormalities. Given the metabolic changes accompanying the loss of abdominal adipose tissue, it is possible that longer follow-up may have demonstrated a benefit with regard to the primary end point. Another imaging study, which will employ measurements of carotid IMT over a longer period of follow-up, may demonstrate a more definitive effect on disease progression.

■ Use of Arterial Wall Imaging in Clinical Practice

- Increasing interest has been focused on the potential role of arterial wall imaging in cardiovascular risk prediction algorithms and in monitoring the effects of treatment in clinical practice.
- Noninvasive imaging (carotid IMT and coronary computed tomography) has been increasingly employed, given its use to associate disease burden and outcome in population studies. No prospective clinical trial has demonstrated that use of imaging alters the management and subsequent outcome of patients.
- Emerging invasive techniques have been proposed to identify vulnerable plaques, with a view to potentially modifying the interventional approach to management. This remains to be tested in clinical trials. Furthermore, pathology studies reveal

that vulnerable plaques rarely occur in isolation within the coronary arterial tree. As a result, it seems likely that systemic approaches to the management of cardiovascular risk will remain the most appropriate course of action.

■ Summary

- Arterial wall imaging has demonstrated that intensive lowering of LDL cholesterol and promoting the biologic activity of HDL cholesterol has a beneficial influence on disease progression.
- Benefits of modifying the ratio of atherogenic to protective lipids are observed across a wide range of the cardiovascular risk spectrum, from the low-risk, asymptomatic patient to the setting of recent acute coronary syndromes.
- Imaging has become an essential tool in the assessment and development of new therapeutic agents that target lipids and lipoproteins.
- Ongoing advances in emerging imaging modalities should permit the ability to evaluate the impact of therapies on the extent, composition, and functional activity of atherosclerotic plaque with high precision in the future.
- The role of arterial wall imaging in the stratification of risk and the triage of patients to the use of preventive medical therapies remains to be defined in randomized clinical trials.

Table 16-1: Summary of Arterial Wall Imaging Modalities

Modality	Invasive	What is imaged	Arterial territories	Comments
Angiography	Yes	Lumen narrowings	Coronary, carotid, peripheral	LDL lowering slows progression; predicts outcome; does not image plaque.
Intimal-medial thickness	No	Early wall changes	Carotid, femoral	Early changes prior to plaque formation. LDL lowering slows progression, predicts outcome.
Intravascular ultrasound	Yes	Full vessel wall and plaque	Coronary, carotid, peripheral	Full extent of atherosclerosis. Targeting LDL and HDL slows disease progression. Developments may characterize plaque components.

Table 16-1:   Continued

Modality	Invasive	What is imaged	Arterial territories	Comments
Computed tomography	No	Lumen, calcium, and with ongoing developments, the potential to image plaque	Coronary	Calcium predicts outcome. Improvements in resolution required to precisely image plaque.
Magnetic resonance	No	Full vessel wall and plaque	Aorta, carotid	Images show extent and composition in large vessels but not in coronaries. Potential for molecular imaging.
Optical coherence tomography	Yes	Fibrous cap	Coronary, carotid, peripheral	Light imaging with high resolution but poor penetration; fibrous cap thickness and inflammatory components of plaque.

■ Suggested Reading

Amarenco P, Labreuche J, Lavallee P, Touboul PJ. Statins in stroke prevention and carotid atherosclerosis: Systematic review and up-to-date meta-analysis. *Stroke*. 2004;35: 2902–2909.

Ballantyne CM. Clinical trial endpoints: Angiograms, events, and plaque instability. *Am J Cardiol*. 1998;82:5M–11M.

Bots ML, Visseren FL, Evans GW, et al. Torcetrapib and carotid intima-media thickness in mixed dyslipidaemia (RADIANCE 2 study): A randomised, double-blind trial. *Lancet*. 2007;370:153–160.

Brown BG, Zhao XQ, Chait A, et al. Simvastatin and niacin, antioxidant vitamins, or the combination for the prevention of coronary disease. *N Engl J Med*. 2001;345:1583–1592.

Crouse JR, 3rd, Raichlen JS, Riley WA, et al. Effect of rosuvastatin on progression of carotid intima-media thickness in low-risk individuals with subclinical atherosclerosis: The METEOR Trial. *JAMA*. 2007;297:1344–1353.

Kalidindi SR, Tuzcu EM, Nicholls SJ. Role of imaging end points in atherosclerosis trials: Focus on intravascular ultrasound. *Int J Clin Pract*. 2007;61:951–962.

Kastelein JJ, Akdim F, Stroes ES, et al. Simvastatin with or without ezetimibe in familial hypercholesterolemia. *N Engl J Med*. 2008;358:1431–1443.

Kastelein JJ, van Leuven SI, Burgess L, et al. Effect of torcetrapib on carotid atherosclerosis in familial hypercholesterolemia. *N Engl J Med*. 2007;356:1620–1630.

Mazzone T, Meyer PM, Feinstein SB, et al. Effect of pioglitazone compared with glimepiride on carotid intima-media thickness in type 2 diabetes: A randomized trial. *JAMA*. 2006;296:2572–2581.

Nicholls SJ, Sipahi I, Schoenhagen P, Crowe T, Tuzcu EM, Nissen SE. Application of intravascular ultrasound in anti-atherosclerotic drug development. *Nat Rev Drug Discov*. 2006;5:485–492.

Nissen SE, Nicholls SJ, Sipahi I, et al. Effect of very high-intensity statin therapy on regression of coronary atherosclerosis: The ASTEROID trial. *JAMA*. 2006;295:1556–1565.

Nissen SE, Nicholls SJ, Wolski K, et al. Comparison of pioglitazone vs glimepiride on progression of coronary atherosclerosis in patients with type 2 diabetes: The PERISCOPE randomized controlled trial. *JAMA*. 2008;299:1561–1573.

Nissen SE, Nicholls SJ, Wolski K, et al. Effect of rimonabant on progression of atherosclerosis in patients with abdominal obesity and coronary artery disease: The STRADIVARIUS randomized controlled trial. *JAMA*. 2008;299:1547–1560.

Nissen SE, Tardif JC, Nicholls SJ, et al. Effect of torcetrapib on the progression of coronary atherosclerosis. *N Engl J Med*. 2007;356:1304–1316.

Nissen SE, Tsunoda T, Tuzcu EM, et al. Effect of recombinant ApoA-I Milano on coronary atherosclerosis in patients with acute coronary syndromes: A randomized controlled trial. *JAMA*. 2003;290:2292–2300.

Nissen SE, Tuzcu EM, Brewer HB, et al. Effect of ACAT inhibition on the progression of coronary atherosclerosis. *N Engl J Med*. 2006;354:1253–1263.

Nissen SE, Tuzcu EM, Libby P, et al. Effect of antihypertensive agents on cardiovascular events in patients with coronary disease and normal blood pressure: The CAMELOT study: A randomized controlled trial. *JAMA*. 2004;292:2217–2225.

Nissen SE, Tuzcu EM, Schoenhagen P, et al. Effect of intensive compared with moderate lipid-lowering therapy on progression of coronary atherosclerosis: A randomized controlled trial. *JAMA*. 2004;291:1071–1080.

Serruys PW, Garcia-Garcia HM, Buszman P, et al. Effects of the direct lipoprotein-associated phospholipase A(2) inhibitor darapladib on human coronary atherosclerotic plaque. *Circulation*. 2008;118:1172–1182.

Tardif JC, Gregoire J, L'Allier PL, et al. Effects of reconstituted high-density lipoprotein infusions on coronary atherosclerosis: A randomized controlled trial. *JAMA*. 2007;297:1675–1682.

Taylor AJ, Kent SM, Flaherty PJ, Coyle LC, Markwood TT, Vernalis MN. ARBITER: Arterial Biology for the Investigation of the Treatment Effects of Reducing Cholesterol: A randomized trial comparing the effects of atorvastatin and pravastatin on carotid intima medial thickness. *Circulation*. 2002;106:2055–2060.

Taylor AJ, Sullenberger LE, Lee HJ, Lee JK, Grace KA. Arterial Biology for the Investigation of the Treatment Effects of Reducing Cholesterol (ARBITER) 2: A double-blind, placebo-controlled study of extended-release niacin on atherosclerosis progression in secondary prevention patients treated with statins. *Circulation*. 2004;110:3512–3517.

Index

Figures and tables are indicated by f and t following the page number.

www.ingramcontent.com/pod-product-compliance
Lightning Source LLC
Chambersburg PA
CBHW070730220326
41598CB00024BA/3373